I0114060

TO YOUR HEALTH
A WORK OF ART
A WORK OF FICTION

MANIFESTING AN EXTRAORDINARY
LIFE AND YOUR DREAMS

BY
JOHN C MILLS MD

Copyright © 2023

All Rights Reserved.

ISBN:

Hardcover: 978-1-917327-48-0

Dedicated To

*All those who dare to Love Unconditionally and Dream
and who have the courage to see their dreams manifest*

and to My Children

Julie, Paige, John, Madison, Hollie

CONTENTS

ABOUT THE AUTHOR

Dr John has a background in Medicine and Health & Wellness—as an Orthopaedic Surgeon, an Emergency Medicine Physician, a Holistic Health Practitioner, a Health Consultant, and a previous Medical Director of two Wellness Centers. He was the Founder of Monadnock Health Resources (for ALL Practitioners of the Healing Arts and Sciences to come together). He also has a background in sports medicine, wilderness medicine, and air-sea rescue, and has had prior certification as a fitness instructor through AAAI/ISMA. Then moving into additional areas of healthy living, John is certified as a 500 Hour Yoga Instructor through Kripalu, and is certified as an Ayurvedic Practitioner through NAMA, committed to generating a health-filled, balanced mind- body-spirit approach to life for all health-conscious human beings. He also dived deeply into the field of energy medicine and explored the path of Shamanism, and now integrates these ancient wisdoms into a balanced holistic healthcare practice.

Dr John sees this path as possible for all human beings through expanded consciousness, knowledge and practice. Simultaneously John is committed to creating a healthy planet by increasing our awareness of, and our relationship with, Nature. As a retired Colonel from the US Army Special Forces, John understands and embodies the warrior spirit—a quality being called for in today's world if we are to survive and thrive as a people . . . as human beings on Planet Earth.

Blending the Best of East and West

PREFACE

The birth of this book is described in the Introduction. What generated that birth will be offered here. My professional background has also been mentioned. What yet needs to be mentioned is what drove the creation of the idea behind the idea. For this I have my patients over many years to thank. Then as I explored other domains of what constitutes healthy living a virtual new world opened to me as to the possibilities. First, I wish to acknowledge all my patients who taught me so much. I still recall faces and names from as far back as medical school.

Much of my early training was about hard work and long hours and dedication to becoming first a physician, then a surgeon, then many years in the Emergency Department where I experienced literally everything of an urgent or emergent nature—and much that was not either, from the point of view of the staff, but from the point of view of the patient there was always the sense of urgency, as this is why they showed up in the Emergency Department in the first place. Many would call their primary care physicians about a health concern and were simply referred to the ER. This perspective and these differing distinctions are important to consider. It was nevertheless true that all of us on staff in the ER were among the frontline providers of emergency care in our hospital system.

And those early days of patient care ushered in my real education in medicine as I later came to regard it. We had an enormous array of available lab tests, radiological studies, and access to an entire hospital staff of physicians for consultation. With time however, I kept having the feeling that something was missing. It wasn't from my patients. It wasn't that time to examine and explain things to my patients wasn't enough. It was, as I was committed to not only taking excellent care of my patients but committed to creating communication and relationship with them that mattered, that I saw as an important part of their care and their recovery from whatever it was. It came down simply to treating my patients like I would like to be treated under similar circumstances. I still believe this and still practice this.

In the ER a good provider must take into consideration the apprehension and fear that is present in most of their patients. I learned to do this fortunately.

One of my middle-of-the-night patients arrived in a lot of distress, complaining of ankle pain without recent injury, crying a lot as she told her story which included a request for pain medication. In the ER we encounter this often, and often it is simply written off as pain medicine-seeking behavior and dismissed. I nevertheless listened to her story of her ankle pain, provided a full Orthopaedic examination of her foot and ankle (which was normal), and then we talked. We had a long conversation that went very well, eventually ending up with us both laughing a lot, and then her going home after hugging each other. She left without any medication—which she no longer felt she needed—as I told her to let me know if she wasn't doing well or needed anything further. And this was sincere, and she knew it. And fortunately it was a relatively slow night in our ER :)

This is yet another example of a way to relate to our patients but possible for all of us to consider. There was an element of humanity and dignity in our interaction, and she taught me so much that night. I wonder if she will recognize our story if she reads this. There are so many stories of little miracles that I experienced in the ER with my patients. . . maybe in another book someday.

What eventually emerged for me however was an experience of a shift in my relationship with some of my colleagues and with some of those in administration. This became over time a significant energy draw and eventually I grew to see my patients were underserved by a system that I saw as disempowering of the very human beings it was designed to serve.

I also came to experience the system as unhealthy for its many hard-working and dedicated HealthCare workers. I will not describe all the details but will say they served to direct me into a deeper search of what contributes to our state of health and an understanding that how we relate and communicate with each other is important to this path.

Hence, I took my first steps in the direction of this deeper inquiry. This journey took me on a path well described in the following pages and opened my eyes to so much more. Much of what I explored became part of my conversations with my patients and it was clear they were open to and aligned with *the more* I was exploring. We had many rich conversations over the years.

This could not be said for many of the professionals I worked with in a hospital setting—physicians, department heads and administrators—who remained largely closed off to this bigger field of discovery and truly caring comprehensively for patients. My patients experienced their own versions of difficulties within the system from their points of view. And when they discovered I was on their side they would open up to me and share more stories.

When I first created a 4-Part program called *Focus on Wellness* after my surgical training was completed and when on staff full time as an Emergency Medicine Physician, I would mention it to some of my ER patients that I would be presenting at a local Sheraton to discuss various aspects of the topic. One General Surgeon (who I had surgically assisted in some of his own surgical cases in my hospital) told me I was a charlatan and a huckster because I was promoting wellness to my ER patients and offering talks locally on wellness, which were not sponsored by the hospital. This experience was a catalyst that sparked a deep concern within me and became a path to my bigger journey ahead.

There were some notable exceptions though, for both physicians and administrators. Some were excellent. The CEO at my first hospital (The Jordan in Plymouth, MA) was extremely supportive of my care and holistic philosophy. When I left there for a position in New Hampshire, he told me there would always be a place for me on his hospital staff if I wanted to return. These were some of the silver linings.

Now enter the second part of this Preface. This too came to me during the night (last night) like so much comes to me as I explain in the book. Fortunately, I listen to what shows up. We all can do this. It is not unique to me. I had to look at what else I really wanted to share with my readers as to why this book was written. Some of this may land well, some may meet with opposition, as it is not part of how our system generally views HealthCare. That is a preparatory statement . . . so prepare yourselves.

You see, I believe our system is in trouble. Actually, I know it is— from my point of view and from the points of view of many of my patients and many professionals in the game whom I have great respect for, some of whom I know personally.

This word *Power* comes up a lot. I used the expression above that patients have become disempowered over the years, so much so because a number of patients whom I've seen tell me that their own physicians would not even listen to them. One told me that her doctor just walked out of the room when she asked a question about an alternative therapy without even discussing it. Is this because we no longer care what our patients have to say to us? Is this driven by fear, the need to control and dominate, not enough time (because we have quotas to meet) the self- absorbed feeling we are right no matter what? It clearly is not driven by love for our work and the feeling it is a privilege to serve (in my opinion).

I know this can be true because it happened to me too, and I'm a physician. More than once a physician did not acknowledge my experience or concerns and simply disregarded both my concerns and my requests. One physician talked about himself and his family and his experience and never even got to my history in any meaningful way. What is all this about?!

The short answer that I have heard expressed over and over again by both patients and HealthCare workers, is that *our system is broken.* Some feel it is beyond repair. I am one of those. I feel these experiences are at the core of the new paradigm emerging that we are

10

all hearing about . . . and *beginning to experience* . . . have been experiencing for some time actually.

This experience of not honoring each other—of not honoring human beings as the magnificent creations we are—is also at the heart of this paradigm shift.

Even as a surgical resident years ago, it wasn't *Mrs. Jones* in Room 304 but the Gall Bladder in 304. We just named parts to identify the patient, in fact, parts that were to be removed or had already been removed. We did not refer to them holistically or with dignity. I noticed this even then.

Where these early experiences were leading me is to the path I followed over the years. That I was experiencing our system as not only disempowering but also as dehumanizing and unhealthy over time was true. More and more became crammed into patient care, longer hours, harder work, more patients to be seen, more rules, more unhappy and discontent colleagues, coupled with a diminishing sense of relationship and purpose within the hospital setting. Something needed to change.

Simultaneously I fully realize the good parts of our system. I often tell my patients about the importance of embracing the best of both worlds—*Blending the Best of East and West*, as my business card states. I tell my patients that if they get run over by a bus in front of our hospital, they could not be in better hands than to be wheeled into my ER or our operating room. And I mean that. How our system manages the chronic stuff is a bigger concern for me. We study disease. We don't study health and wellness. Although that too is happening.

Fast forward to today. We are all becoming increasingly aware of our system and of those behind it that drive how patient care shows up to each of us. We are all becoming more aware of the unhealthy aspects of our HealthCare system. What can we do about this?

My journey eventually took the form of this book in addition to my many pauses along the way to explore life at its many levels. I still maintain an office and see patients who desire a consultation with me. I created a few pages of my background that I now share with

HealthCare Providers here on Kauai as well as anyone interested in a consultation, just to give them a clearer picture of my background and what I offer. This will be in the Appendix area. I think it is useful for all of us in HealthCare to begin making up our practices in a way that truly speaks to us, fulfills our personal dreams as to why we began walking this path in the first place, and to assess if we are truly serving our patients. I call this part of the Reinvention process as we each bring healthier changes to our profession and to the field of HealthCare.

This is what contributed to the creation of *TO YOUR HEALTH . . . A WORK OF ART . . . A WORK OF FICTION*. My intention was simply to deliver more awareness of this power that we all possess of taking better care of ourselves, of putting back into our own hands, and our own hearts and minds really, that which will serve us more ideally. Everything shared in my book is true and I have experienced it as written. I eventually realized there was great value in each of us becoming more aware of the power we each hold within ourselves. I believe we each have access to all the answers we need to heal, recover, flourish, and thrive, but there is a learning curve in accessing this knowledge (or *knowing* as I call it).

I also believe it is possible to manifest our dreams whatever they may be without limitation—another learning curve perhaps but all mentioned in the book and all within our ability to embrace and experience. Many already have. This is just about sharing more of the wealth.

So, each of you will have to decide if this journey is worth taking or not (for a lifetime hopefully). I have experienced it as a deep journey for me, both within and without, for my life as well as in writing this book. It is a relatively short read. I used to describe it to my friends that would ask what it was about. I would just say it was about becoming as healthy as you wish to be, and about realizing your dreams.

Then I began saying it was about *YOU*, each of you (whoever I was speaking to), in any way you choose to live your life . . . and realize your dreams whatever they may be. Recently I have been just saying *This is your Roadmap to Bliss . . . and manifesting your dreams without limitation.*

ACKNOWLEDGMENTS

First and foremost, my five children—Julie, Paige, John, Madison, Hollie—who provided an experience of family love and support and inspiration which allowed me to even consider the scope of this endeavor, so supportive throughout all this and affording this to be a joyful undertaking.

I also shared my thoughts and writing with more than a few friends, and some close friends, who also encouraged me along this journey. They include Jitka Robinson, a very close friend since our Yoga and Ayurveda training days at Kripalu, and the inspiration behind my poem, *When Old Souls Touch*, who has agreed to illustrate one of my future books on children; Edith Shamrell, a close friend and Yogi who brought her magic from Barcelona and who shared her experience with me of *MY* unseen world, who is also walking a Shaman's path; Kim Wood, a close friend and the other magician with me *together apart* in the poem *Moonshadow*, and always so full of encouragement and excitement; Carolina Vasquez, originally from Ecuador. Meet her in the poem *Journey to the North*—my Shaman partner in that direction. Carolina's whole family has welcomed me into their home anytime I am in Canada—her home is my home, as she put it. Thank you Caro, Mike, Miriam (her Mom), Danalia & Aralia (her daughters); Shanon & Marv Hardwood, my Shaman teachers in the Kimmapii School of Shamanism and Elders in the First Nations Blackfoot tribe, that contributed so much to my training and my journey; Supriya Shanbhag, a close friend and new member of our Kimmapii Community who just completed her training in the Shaman's Altar and was the inspiration behind several of my poems; Leilani Levesque, a close friend and member of my Shaman community, and one of the Goddesses in Voices of the Goddess; Alanna Golden, my *sister* from Brazil (now in Cusco) who has walked paths with me in the past and continues to do so; Kazumi Sakurai, my new friend and a professional photographer who intends to capture the divine in all her images; Michael Shooltz, a bright light in our Kaua'i Ohana who generously shares wisdom, his music, and himself with us all; Dennis Mendonca and Ken Jopling and Tom Cobb, who share the sacred magic of Riversong with so many; Steve 'Stream' Backinoff and Maronda, and all the dancers and musicians for Dances of Universal Peace at our gatherings; Raevon White, a close friend from our Shaman training together, endlessly kind and supportive; Linda Kodnar, another Canadian friend and voice of encouragement for my book; Kat Roberts (Nova), one of the Wisdom Weavers who shared long walks and deep talks with me; Katie Johnson, an inspiration to my work during our walks with her dog, Grif, and her husband Garrett, who provided timely needed assistance with my communications with ADP; and my very good friend, Flip Cordova, who knows the island like the back of his hand, and with whom I have had many great conversations.

My son John whose words show up under the chapter on Family--his journey and the strength of his commitment to his path are an inspiration to all young men; Joya and DeShaya, who know who they are and what they contribute.

The Goddesses in Voices of the Goddess . . . Ilona Drost, Dayna Catt, Shanon Harwood, Paige Mills (my daughter), Jitka Robinson, Edith Shamrell, Julie Mills (my daughter), Madison Mills (my daughter), Alana Agustin, Kazumi Sakurai, Alanna Golden, and Leilani Levesque.

There is also Kripalu, its teachers and staff, and my classmates, many of whom I got to think of as family when I studied there—a place I came to call my home away from home.

There are some paddlers at Kukui'ula Outrigger Canoe Club who enjoyed the ocean with me in an outrigger (some were part of my original 6-man racing crew) and each of whom shared the Ohana spirit of Kauai with me, which thus related and contributed to the creation of this book. They include Pancho, Rob, Kerry, Jack, Gavin, Gary, Tom, Teva, Coach Laola, as well as Meghan, Leah, Ratih, Michele, and Ashley. Whether intended or not by the cover artist, the image at the bottom of the cover of this book is the silhouette of Kauai as seen from sea, a portion of that view we often experienced from our canoes. I did not suggest this as part of the cover design. There is indeed magic here.

I must also include all my many patients who taught me over the years that a better way was necessary, my teachers and the writers and authors and artists whom I've encountered that led by example and by their words and art (some of whom appear in this book), and all those in the unseen world who have accompanied me on this journey, and the many friends not mentioned here but part of my journey.

I would be amiss to not mention all my friends and shop keepers at the Warehouse in Lawai, Kauai, where I have spent many hours writing at one of their tables, occasionally sipping delicious coffee from Kind Koffee inside the Warehouse. The baristas there are owner Taeru, Tapa, Briana, Courtney, Niah, and Beigh. Other shop owners who have now become part of my Kauai family include: Robin McCoy and Shelagh Balmores (Art Gallery & Studio); Melissa & Kevin Roxburgh (The Island Beet); Maren Arismendez-Herrera and Alfred Herrera and Shannon Lorenzo (Sugar Skull); Jacqueline & Jake Schmidt & Lauren Weber (Wildflower Boutique and Drift Microbar Kauai and Navydylan); Taylor & Shannan Morgan at Navydylan; Laurie Hutchinson and Nadine Robinson (Lily Koi); Kathryn Ledesma and Debra (Aphrodite's Treasures); Maui and Jody Kjeldsen and Kai Kealoha of Hanako (Maui made my two outrigger canoe paddles, a true craftsman and legendary paddler); Trysen Kaneshige (Inspire to Create Media); Eric Cano (island clothing at *iamislander.com*), and Erwin Cano (3D Artist for I am islander). If ever on the South Shore of Kauai, do not miss the Warehouse and all the shop owners and their employees and the locals who frequent this place. They have each shared in my journey at the Warehouse engaged in all their own projects of creativity.

16

I only just met a new person at Amazon Digital Publishing, but I sense I will be working closely with her and the team responsible for getting my book out there in the world, so I will thank them now. So far, the players and my experience with ADP have changed a bit. I will update these acknowledgements at the time of publication for accuracy. I anticipate a long and exciting relationship with my team at Amazon Digital Publishing if things go as planned.

I submitted my idea, my vision, for an attractive cover design, but it was the design team and artists that gave life to that idea. I wanted the earth in it, symbolizing the beauty of Gaia and the importance of my relationship with Gaia. I wanted the sky around Earth deepening into space and stars symbolizing the vastness yet perceived proximity of all the grandeur that surrounds our Earth within all this vastness. And I wanted the title to draw attention. The addition of Kaua'i and the ocean below the image of Earth was an amazing touch, and not suggested by me. Kaua'i is dear to my heart, and the artist knew that. All was delivered in the captivating form before you—so beautiful. And lastly, the Editorial Review *got me* exactly, got exactly what I wished to convey to my readers. This revealed great promise that perhaps this work would reach others in a deep and meaningful way, my intention from the start.

Thank you all who contributed for your hard work and dedication in bringing this creation and my dream to all my readers. I suspect we will work together again.

In my Shamanic traditions of Plains Native American and that of the Q'ero of Peru it is both appropriate and important to acknowledge all the assistance and input from Creator, from all Spirits of Earth and beyond, *all my relations*, my ancestors, Mother Earth (Pachamama), Father Sun, Grandmother Moon, and all Star Nations. Ho!

Thank You All

John Mills

FOREWARD

Introduction to the Foreword

Dear Readers, I am experimenting with a variation of the usual way a Foreward is written for a book. Usually it is composed by someone who the author asks to review the book, and optimally someone of some notoriety who is known to many readers, as this adds to its universal appeal, presumably.

I tried this approach. I reached out to a few well-known personalities and successful writers who published books. I am a new writer. This is my first book. No one responded except one, who agreed to perhaps endorse it but whose schedule was too busy to write a Foreward—totally understandable. Most very well-known people are too busy to engage in this extra work.

And then the editorial staff at Amazon Digital Publications stepped up and provided an Editorial Review, part of their agreement with me when signing on. No name was attached to this review, but it was clearly from my team supporting my book being published. When I read it, it brought tears to my eyes. I realized whoever wrote that *totally got me!* They captured exactly what I wished to convey to my readers all over the world. And it was not written by me. I felt so honored and seen. I would be so appreciative if the author of this review at ADP would put their name on it, but I am no less appreciative if they don't. My highest gratitude for a beautiful rendition of what my book is about. Thank you. And now . . .

Editorial Review by Sabrina Miller at ADP
As The Foreword

"To Your Health: A Work of Art, A Work of Fiction" is a literary masterpiece that weaves together the intricacies of life, love, and healing in a mesmerizing tapestry of words. This enchanting book opens its pages with an enthralling Chapter One, inviting readers on an introspective journey of self-discovery, empowerment, and the profound nuances of human existence. The author's eloquent prose and deeply philosophical tone create an immersive experience that transcends traditional storytelling. From the very first lines, readers are transported into a shamanic perspective of time, challenging linear notions of beginnings and endings. This unique lens empowers readers to embrace the idea that their journey can unfold in unexpected ways, at any point. The opening chapter sets the stage for a captivating reading adventure that celebrates individuality and the intricate beauty of life's intricate design. A standout feature of this chapter is the author's reverence for the diversity of human experience. With an unwavering respect for the uniqueness of each life, the author reminds us that there are as many paths to fulfillment as there are people. This inclusivity not only honors individuality but also imparts the invaluable lesson that there is no single blueprint for life's journey.

Throughout the chapter, the author gently guides readers to step away from societal norms and external influences, urging them to embrace the vast terrain of their inner selves. This shift towards self-exploration approached with a beginner's mind, forms the foundation for growth and transformation. The concept of two SELVES – the everyday self and the expansive BIG SELF – encourages readers to delve into the depths of their consciousness and intuition, transcending the boundaries of the ordinary.

The chapter elegantly introduces intuition as a bridge connecting the individual with the divine. The author's emphasis on the richness of intuitive experiences is particularly captivating, elevating the

19

reader's awareness beyond imagination to a profound connection with cosmic intelligence. By encouraging readers to discern between mental noise and intuitive wisdom, the author empowers them to tap into their innate wellspring of insight. The author's mastery of these ideas shines through, creating a dialogue that is accessible and enlightening. The interweaving of personal experiences, including the author's journey as a certified Yoga Instructor, infuses authenticity and depth into the narrative, making esoteric notions relatable and applicable to readers' lives. In essence, these early chapters serve as a transformative gateway to self-discovery, intuition, and empowerment. It beckons readers to release preconceived notions, embark on their own unique journeys of exploration, and choose paths that resonate profoundly with their innermost desires. The wisdom shared is not imposed as doctrine but extended as an invitation to uncover the truth for oneself. These early chapters stand also as a testament to the author's ability to craft prose that not only informs but also inspires and guides, setting a luminous tone for what promises to be an illuminating and enlightening literary journey.

All chapters captivate from the very beginning, immersing readers in a profound exploration of self-discovery and empowerment. With a blend of wisdom, vulnerability, and optimism, the author's words resonate deeply, igniting a spark of hope within every reader. The theme of embracing life's potential is explored with profound insight, underscoring the interconnectedness of all beings and the transformative power within each individual to shape their own reality.

The author's candid reflections on personal experiences forge an authentic and relatable connection with readers. Through stories of trials, growth, and transformation, the author encourages us to shed the limitations of old narratives and embrace the prospect of reinvention. This call for change and personal development resonates universally, sparking a desire for a similar journey of self-discovery. What sets this section apart is the seamless integration of practical advice and spiritual wisdom. The concept of storytelling as a tool for empowerment is particularly captivating. Moreover, the author's candid account of surrendering to a higher power, to Spirit, showcases vulnerability as a source of strength and highlights the profound impact of releasing the ego. This transition from ego-driven pursuits to a more holistic, connected existence resonates deeply with readers.

As the author delves into the concept of manifestation, co-creation with the universe is vividly depicted. The idea that we can actively participate in the "manufacture" of our desires by collaborating with a guiding force evokes curiosity and wonder. The author's personal journey of book writing as a manifestation process adds authenticity, forging a powerful synergy between their words and lived experiences. The interplay of introspection, spiritual insight, and practical guidance renders this section an engaging read for anyone seeking to unlock their potential and transform their lives. The author's genuine enthusiasm and encouragement invite readers to become active architects of their own journeys, urging them to reflect, rewrite, and reconstruct the narratives that shape their reality.

The engaging writing style bridges the gap between complex concepts and readers from diverse backgrounds. The author's willingness to share personal experiences and insights lend authenticity to the narrative, forging a deep connection between the content and the reader. A distinguishing element of this book excerpt is the emphasis on simplicity and mindfulness. The call to approach healing with intention, patience, and gentleness underscores the significance of self-awareness and introspection. This perspective resonates, inspiring readers to embark on their own healing journeys with open hearts and minds.

The incorporation of references to Ayurvedic principles and ancient wisdom adds depth and credibility to the discourse. These references enrich the narrative by presenting diverse viewpoints that extend beyond modern medical paradigms, inviting readers to embrace a holistic approach to well- being. Moreover, the exploration of the relationship between nourishment and healing – encompassing both physical and emotional aspects – illuminates the profound impact of our choices on overall health. This provides readers with a practical framework for making mindful decisions that contribute positively to their healing processes.

A notable strength of this book is its ability to provoke introspection and contemplation. By posing questions and encouraging readers to explore their own perspectives, the author facilitates an interactive reading experience that transcends passive engagement. The narrative seamlessly transitions between personal reflections, philosophical contemplation, and practical suggestions, sustaining reader engagement and investment.

What truly shines in one of the chapters is the author's passionate call for change. The author proposes a paradigm shift towards healthier family dynamics and improved communication, underscoring the importance of listening to children. The commitment to inspiring transformation on both an individual and global level is palpable, making it difficult not to join in the quest for positive change. The inclusion of a heartfelt contribution from the author's own son adds an extra layer of authenticity and relatability. This personal touch reinforces the notion that the book is not a monologue, but rather a communal effort to foster understanding, growth, and harmony in the world.

In summary, the book is an uplifting and thought-provoking exploration of family, childhood, and the power of positive transformation. Combining personal anecdotes, philosophical contemplation, and practical suggestions, the author adeptly guides readers on a journey of reflection, transformation, and a renewed appreciation for the significance of familial bonds.

Editorial Review by Sabrina Miller, ADP

Sabrina Miller

INTRODUCTION

To Your Health, A Work of Art, A work of Fiction, was born years ago. It arrived in the form of a dream. The time has arrived to share it. *To Your Health* is a toast, a toast to our health, whatever that may be for any one of us. Toasting has a celebratory note—that it is within each of us to enhance, enrich, embrace, and celebrate the essence of who we are. It also speaks to manifesting our dreams, for those of us who dream . . . *and we all dream.*

As a physician I have spent most of my professional career considering what constitutes health, and specifically, what exists beyond good health, beyond just the absence of disease—what may possibly exist in the realm of superior health, of extraordinary vitality, energy, and a sense of extreme wellbeing. I have spent far more time engaged in the inquiry than in discovering answers or solutions. This inquiry keeps me open to possibility. That said, patterns of health and successful healthy living have emerged. This I will share with you in the pages of this book.

First, I want to tell each and every one of you, ***do not believe a word of what I say***. That is not to say that there is no truth in what I say, as perhaps there is, but I want each of you to discover that truth for yourselves. If anything fits and feels right as to what is said, then try implementing it in the test tube called your life and see how it works. Prove it is true for you, that it works, or simply discard it. It is my sincere hope that some of it will prove of value to you in your life and sticks, but I am not attached to that. And I would not be presenting a lifetime of work to you if I did not believe in it.

My ideas may come across to you as strange, unbelievable, without merit or scientific proof. That's okay. That's where the *fiction* part of the title comes in. *You see, I'm making it all up.* Treat all this as pure fiction if you wish and if that makes it easier to assimilate and process, like a novel, perhaps like a good novel, and discover the entertainment in it. The Truth is however, this is all true, all my experiences as recorded, and just as I stated in the Preface. This book is Non-Fiction although to some of you readers it may appear fictitious. That will be up for each of you to decide. For me, it all happened as stated, even the crazy-sounding parts. I have discovered life can be playful, fun, creative and a joy to experience, or not.

Since I have experienced the *'or not'* a lot in my life, as well as the fun and joy and play, I wholeheartedly recommend the fun and play and joyful times. I have also noticed that these experiences—of fun, play and joy—are related to good health and happiness. The trick is for us to discover what this means for each of us and then implement it in our lives and see what shows up.

And now for the *Art* part of the title—*A Work of Art.* Life and living are to be sure forms of art. This does not need to be seen as such but just consider it. What I am suggesting is that we become artists in the creation of our own life, and not just any artist, but a great and accomplished painter, sculptor, musician, poet, writer, teacher, athlete—you name it, whatever artist you wish to be—and then allow the canvas, or the page, or the chunk of clay, or the music, or any endeavor that you are working with, to express YOU in the best and most artistic form of expression that you can come up with. This becomes a creative challenge for a lifetime.

What may facilitate experiencing your life as a work of art, as a work of fiction, is discarding a commonly held misconception— *buying into consensual reality.* The bad news is most of us buy into consensual reality and many of us are not even aware of it. The good news is we don't have to.

What is consensual reality? It is the notion that we should do whatever everyone else thinks is best for us, whether it's our parents shortly after we become aware of what they say when we are very young, or the school system and our teachers, or the church, the news, TV, magazines, the internet... .In short it is every bit of information that is out there that is imposed upon our thoughts of who we are and who we should be in order to show up successfully in life. In this view we need to blindly accept what we experience from others as the truth—as what we need to know, say, do, think, be, to be accepted or belong, to fit in.

Do you know who Don Miguel Ruiz is? He is the author of *The Four Agreements and The Voice of Knowledge*, among his books. In addition to his being a writer, he is an MD and a surgeon, and a Shaman of the Toltec lineage. In his *Voice of Knowledge*, he states there are only two rules: One is to not believe anything that anyone tells you, i.e. consensual reality; the other is to not believe yourself, because each of us have bought into consensual reality—the words and advice of others—and that is what we think we know, and not what we actually know. This book is about getting in touch with what we actually know to free us up to be extraordinary and creative human beings with the capacity to live amazing lives.

Speaking of health, we will visit together what health may be, may look like, and we will notice it may be very different for each of us. We will explore together what we think constitutes good health and healthy living, and most importantly, what may lie way beyond our beliefs of what we perceive as good health and vitality.

In our western tradition, health for many people means the absence of disease. In the ancient wisdom of **Ayurveda** (Ayurveda is translated as the *science of life*, or *life knowledge*), the Ayurvedic definition of health is more descriptive (appearing in Chapter 15). We will look at which definition serves us best, or better yet, create our own to meet the needs of the life we are designing. We will also explore the choices we make in creating a healthy and fulfilling life— and whether those choices are working for us. I appreciate that some of us may not want to be healthy, or more accurately, may not want to put the effort into becoming healthy.

The word *effort* is worth discussing. Many people who feel that if anything is worth doing that is big, successful, accomplishes a lot, think that it requires a lot of work and takes great effort to get there. I would like to suggest the notion that we may be able to accomplish much through *effortless ease*. This idea came to me a long time ago while musing on why do things need to be difficult to accomplish when they also seem so important to living life well? It wasn't until years later while reading a book by Deepak Chopra that he used that exact same expression—that we can accomplish great things through effortless ease.

The more I accepted this principle, the more I incorporated it into my life and soon I noted there was truth in it. I also noticed others speaking of it, people appearing very successful with their lives and accomplishments. And truthfully, simplicity has always appealed to me. *Effortless ease* has a ring of simplicity to it. If I can do something simply, I prefer that.

So, I will endeavor to bring my thoughts to you as simply as I can. Even simple, you will discover there is much to do, know, understand as you explore your SELVES, *but within the background of effortless ease* in your life's perspective, perhaps it may not feel like a difficult process. *It just becomes 'an is', 'a something to discover and work with'*, without the added baggage of how tough it may appear. It may even become an exciting adventure for you, one that you can't wait to dive into.

How many people do you know who have done it the hard way? I have, many times, and it taught me to look deeper.

What I will ask of you is simply to be open to possibilities, maintain an inquisitive mind, and be willing to experiment with yourself and with life. And then start noticing what is showing up.

Oh, and a few words about fun. Fun isn't talked about so much. We have become serious human beings—*human doings* more accurately. Just look around and see what is there, in your family, your friends, your work, your life. If fun is showing up a lot, you are on the right track. If it isn't, look deeper and perhaps become the creator of this quality in your own life. Fun goes hand-in-hand with joy, play, laughter, levity. And by the way, I have discovered it has a lot to do with our state of health and our overall enjoyment of our lives. More on this later.

And there is another quality which I have discovered is very important to good health and contentment—*Love*. I think of love in many ways: Love is cosmic glue. It is an energy and a force that is available to all humans, all beings, all of life. This is my view. You may consider it for yourself. I believe love itself is intelligent.

To the degree of our awareness and usage of this energy we can bring it into our every moment to positive effect and benefit to ourselves and others and for our whole planet. Each of us are gifted with this ability and this capacity to love, and I believe it is different and unique for each of us. More will be said about this later. This is only to consider for deeper exploration in later chapters.

So, this is a glimpse at the journey before you. It is not required that you take it. It is simply an offering of something that has the possibility—perhaps the probability—of transforming your life. That is the challenge. I have five children and when they were young, we always called any new experience a *Bilbo Baggins adventure* (Lord of the Rings). They are grown up now and we still refer to our new experiences or challenges that show up as a Bilbo Baggins adventure.

Welcome to your personal Bilbo Baggins adventure! :)

. . .

John Mills

PART I
THE JOURNEY OF
DISCOVERY

THE JOURNEY OF DISCOVERY

Introduction to Part I

We are all in the process of discovering. We all have an idea of who we are. This journey is about the discovery of much deeper parts of Our Selves, the discovery of that which may be hidden beneath the surface for each of us but is available to each of us when we explore deeper, or when we simply look and listen.

Each chapter was a gift to me as I was writing, and so I pass it on to each of you as a gift. What you do with the gifts contained within is up to you. My intention is that it be a grand and rich discovery and exactly what you are looking for in your lives.

Let the Journey begin . . .

John Mills

Chapter 1
THE JOURNEY AND CHOICE
OF PATH

Let's start at the beginning, which can be anywhere. A shamanic perspective is that time is a circle—not linear—hence there is no beginning point, no end point. It just depends upon where you jump in. Let's pick a place to jump in together.

This book is about health, and my intention is that it be personal and about our own health—about what it is to experience life in our own bodies with whatever we came with. So, as many humans as there are in existence at this moment is exactly the number of ways to experience life—for humans. No one size fits all. We are all unique beings and this book will explore discovering that uniqueness, appreciating our individual uniqueness, and what we may each discover to become our own dream fulfillment.

How do we best accomplish this? I believe it will be optimal for us to acknowledge our past, let go of it, let go of the consensual reality that has ruled over us, and discover what knowing our SELVES can really mean for us. We all possess great power but many of us are unaware of it. Or if aware, we may need some guidance as to how to use it most effectively as we steer our ships, sometimes in calm waters, sometimes in turbulent seas.

One way to begin this journey into exploration of the *SELF* is to clear our minds of all notions that we know anything. Adopt a beginner's mind. Or become the infant you once were when you entered the world and all was new, and nothing was consciously known at the time before the influence of the outside world took over and dictated how we should show up. You just simply *were*—in a state of beingness. This is a very fertile state for growth.

There are many paths to health, happiness, and enlightenment. You only have to choose one—your path. And if you don't, one will happen for you. There is always a path. The important part is that maybe you consciously reflect on which one you want to walk for your life. Choosing your own path makes the journey so much more fulfilling and rewarding. It is said we all have a future. It is also said not all of us have a destiny. Unless perhaps you know your destiny . . . or perhaps you become aware that you can create one.

Creating your own destiny will be discussed later in this book, in case you don't have one and decide you do want one—makes the journey more interesting perhaps, maybe not, but it definitely ups your awareness in life once you identify why you came. And this heightened awareness contributes to how you participate. Your choice though. You'll be fine without a destiny . . . probably :)

Let's examine our SELF first. It's good to acknowledge the SELF and then get to know it before asking it what it wants in this lifetime. Consider there are two SELVES, one is our *little self*, also known as our ordinary reality—just our little me, our little body, our little mind, and our little very contained and very restricted experience of our little life. That is not to disparage that aspect of who we think we are. We each have that—all of us human beings—but there is so much more.

That's where our *BIG SELF* comes in. Some of you have heard of this and some of you haven't. It's not new with me either. I didn't originate the idea. It's been around a long, long time. Remember I told you not to believe a word I say. But I've encountered this idea so much over most of my years that I'm passing it on to you because I finally accepted it with my emerging beginner's mind. The notion has value. It is simply that we are much greater than meets the eye—and the ears, nose, taste, touch—all our senses. They really inform us so little about our world, our unseen world. Some of you may have experienced this and some of you may have yet to do so. This book will be about the journey we each can take into the unseen world.

This is a good introduction to the importance of family and community. In family and community, these ideas get batted around sometimes, maybe shared, and discussed. They are often passed down from the elders, literally a dying breed— not just because they are older but because they are not paid as much attention to as in earlier years. In some cultures, they are still honored and listened to—not so much in ours. If you have an elder in your life that you love and honor and respect, hold onto her or him as long as possible. Pure Gold

There will be much said about family later. Let's get back to the SELF. What does your SELF want out of life? This may be a very complex question but let's approach it more simply at first. Remember, simple is good.

On most people's lists are good health and happiness. That is what most selfs will say when asked, although the list can vary widely in responses.

This is a good first question to consider. What do you want for your Self for this life? I will not answer for you since I don't know. Consider this homework before you proceed to the next chapter. Really examine what you want in life. And how will you know when you have it? Will there be an endpoint, a destination, a signpost, an image of what it will look like, or feel like, when you've attained what you set as your benchmark?

Or maybe, there's nothing out there on your radar? For you it may be all about the journey, and nothing about the destination. This will be for you to decide. Both will be discussed further, but most important, you have a say in the matter. It is your life and you get to choose how you wish to live it. This seems obvious but you would be surprised at how many of us allow others to make these decisions for us, to dictate how we should live our life. We talked about this already. Be ever present to the stealthy and invasive nature of consensual reality.

You see, just knowing about consensual reality warns us to look out for its influence and effect on our lives. That's enough. Now just practice not being controlled or influenced by it for the rest of your life. You'll get better at it as you practice. Pretty soon you will not settle for anything less than what you've made up about your own life, and then live as you desire. Simple, isn't it?

So, to summarize: Pick a path . . . identify your desires and dreams, consider your destiny, talk to your SELF about it, and don't let anyone adversely influence you (consensual reality) in how you wish to live. There are some rules, natural laws, ways of being, that are best to be subscribed to. We will talk about consequences for not following natural laws in the pages ahead.

To be more thorough, we should discuss some ways of talking to our Self first after distinguishing which Self we are talking with, and then learn some ways of listening. Some of you may be very adept at listening—and some may be novices, or just think you are good listeners. Let's all pretend we are beginners at listening, the **Beginner's Mind** notion. This is the fertile soil I referred to before that is optimal for growing.

First distinguish between higher self and the lower self—big S or little s. If you haven't heard of this distinction, begin to familiarize your Self with the notion that both exist. Little self is sometimes known as ordinary reality, moment to moment flow of thoughts—the monkey mind—always chattering, never quieting down, always with an opinion of what you should do, what you didn't do, what you haven't done enough of, what he said, what she said, and on and on and on. **This is an example of monkey mind**—nonstop stuff that runs through our minds every day. There is little of substantial value or contribution to life and living. We get bored quickly and in fact it keeps us from really living, if we pay attention to what is happening. And we've all been there.

This is why we hear so much about the value of meditation, finding stillness, being in Nature, learning to quiet or calm the monkey mind. Yoga is one such method. *"Yogas chitti vritti narodaha*—Yoga causes the cessation of mind chatter."* Yoga means connecting the mind and the body—to yoke the two together. These practices are now getting us into the realm of the Higher Self, a realm of expanded consciousness, heightened awareness, of connection to a vast unseen world of possibilities and experiences . . . and of a deeper connection with your SELF. Many have experienced this. I have too. In fact, we all have but only for glimpses for some, with not full awareness of what is happening. But don't believe me. Find out for yourself. Explore, experiment, enrich, by trying some paths that have been meaningful for many. I won't say trust me . . . but what the heck . . . trust me :)

I teach Yoga. I am a certified Yoga Instructor 500-Hour RYT. I have often asked my classes over time, "How many here have done Yoga before?" Hands go up. Then I ask, how many of you have practiced yoga for say longer than 6 months?" Some hands go down and a number remain up. I then ask, "For those who have been doing Yoga for a while, how many feel their practice has transformed their life?" The same hands stay up and some of the less-than-6-month group go up. Maybe a clue.

For those new at Yoga or whose hands aren't up, they get a glimpse that maybe this is a good thing. If Yoga isn't for you, that's okay. Find something else that gets you out of bed in the morning and gets your juices flowing—something that causes the cessation of mind chatter, perhaps even brings you a little joy.

So now we understand the distinction between monkey mind and calm mind, between lower, very busy, everyday reality self, and still, calm, heightened consciousness and expanded awareness SELF. The distinction becomes clearer with practice so don't worry if this isn't clear yet.

The important thing to consider is that when you begin talking to your Self, be sure that you are talking to your higher Self. The information shared is richer and more substantial. The same is true for when you are listening—listen to your higher SELF. We're not done with this topic so just stay tuned.

This brings us into the realm of intuition. Most everyone is familiar with this word. To become familiar with the experience is another matter altogether. Simply stated, your intuition is your connection to the divine, to Source, to all that is. When we have a sense of something, a gut-feeling, a knowing, for any reason, that isn't our ordinary mind chatter talking at us. This is the door opening to our intuitive world.

Some call this door opening experience talking to our Higher Self, to Cosmic Intelligence, to Source, to God, to Spirit, to Creator—you can call it whatever you like. It is not the label of the experience, but the experience itself. It is not the knowledge of it, but in the knowing of it. It is not based on facts or science. It is simply a knowing. If anyone has experienced an intuitive hit or gut-feeling, or their sixth sense, they know what I'm talking about. If they then acted on that intuition, they may have noticed the action taken was of value to their life, to the lives of others perhaps.

The question was asked during my Shamanic training in the Medicine Wheel—the Shaman's Altar, "What If it's just my imagination?" Our teacher and mentor, a Shaman of many years, Marv Harwood, replied, "Your imagination is like talking to God."

How can you tell if you are talking to God or if it is just your Monkey mind chattering away in its usual constant mode? . . . because of the quality of the communication, the message, the simplicity of it, the absence of consensual reality (the voices of many) intruding. Don't worry, you get more adept at it with practice. Soon you can listen and sort out the junk mail in just a moment or two. Following through on your intuition and taking action, if called for, can happen anytime you choose.

So what's the value in this experience of intuition? That is for you to decide. I have felt it, and found it of great value, and so I pass it on to you. I am certainly not the originator of this experience, and many can speak to its value, even in saving lives at times. So explore it, practice it. See what shows up—perhaps there will be some examples later in these pages. No stone left unturned in our exploration together into health.

Oh, and why does this topic of intuition show up in Chapter 1 about our journey and choosing our path? It is because our intuition can be useful in uncovering our path. Just ask your Self and see what comes back. The trick is to trust that first impression, that is your spark of genius speaking to you, your shaman within, your personal guru speaking to you, your connection to Source. Listen closely. It'll get better with practice.

The problem for most of us is we see through muddy waters. Our systems are polluted. We have toxic build-up and residue since shortly after birth. Most of us may not eat an optimal diet to keep our systems clean. Add to that all the mental and emotional debris that accumulates over time—and which we do not let go of— and that too muddies the water and makes it harder to see clearly.

Then there are those of us who have been damaged and seem to express the effects of that in our lives, via deceit and dishonesty, betrayal, cheating, stealing, taking anything that is not ours, manipulation of others, domination and control issues, anger, greed, blame, shame, guilt, jealousy and envy, abuse of others or self, and crimes against nature and humanity, and worse. You can name more. All of these are qualities of being human, and probably all, or most of us, have been there and experienced these qualities, and maybe inflicted them upon others.

These are all just experiences and although one can attach a rightness or wrongness to them, that is not the point. The point is to learn from them. You have maybe heard the expression, *there are no mistakes, only learning experiences.* Life is a learning experience. We can learn quickly or take ages, even lifetimes, to get the message, to mine the gold, to discover the silver lining of the dark cloud.

I will state that the cleaner we become through and through, the more the mud turns to clear water, the quicker we get to see more clearly that which we are to see, the grandeur and the miraculous of life, the possibility of each life. If you've been badly damaged in life, this may not be apparent at this time. In that case just consider it then—it may take on a different appearance later. And remember, don't believe a word I say. Try it out for yourself and see what shows up.

Chapter 2
THE PATH CHOSEN, NOW WHAT

In chapter One we looked at choosing a path. For those of us who aren't clear on our path, or haven't a clue how to choose one, that's okay. Welcome to the human race! You have lots of company. Choosing a path is good to do because it may add clarity and direction to your life, affects future choices. That said, it is fine if you take any path while considering what you want to do when you grow up. I'm still growing up but feel I've settled into a path largely of my design, have seen my destiny, and that colors my experience of life. It also influences me a bit as to how I show up in the world. I can change this anytime. I choose not to at this time. And I'm not done yet.

Too often our path is chosen by others, parents, teachers, even friends with strong influence—even the military in the days of the draft. It would be great if we could just thank them for sharing and move on in our own unique way. We don't usually do this. We listen to many cues and clues of others of what we should become in life.

The Sanskrit word for our life's purpose is dharma—the reason we were born to this lifetime. Deepak Chopra has expressed in his writing that we each possess a unique talent, an ability, that we alone can deliver to the world better than anyone else. I believe this too. We are all unique. That is, when we are steeped in our dharma, our life's purpose, and are aligned with that purpose, we then embark upon a unique path to manifest this purpose in the world. It is also said that Spirit lines up behind us and supports us on that path. You can consider this assertion. I am not the first one to say it. It could be true. You'll have to find out for yourself.

Sometimes we set out on a path not knowing why we chose it, or where it may eventually lead. When I went to college, I had a notion that I may go on to medical school with no good understanding how that came about. There were no doctors in my family. My mother was a registered nurse. My father was in education. There was no push in my family for me to become a doctor, no pressure at all. I was an only child. And there I was heading off to college with this idea that I might become a doctor.

The only other thing I was drawn to consider was becoming a fighter pilot. I also had no idea why this drew me in, as there were no family members that I knew who were pilots. In fact, I was the only one in my family who served in the military that I was aware of. While I jumped out of a number of planes during most of my career with Special Forces, I never flew anything other than a single engine fixed wing aircraft, and second seat in a helicopter, hardly a fighter pilot experience. This military story will be further explained later pertinent to our conversation of dharma.

Like so many people starting out in life, we seem to fall onto a path, and not be conscious of choosing one, certainly for many of us not realizing our dharma at the tender young ages we typically start out at in life. This is where I believe the element of trust enters the equation. I don't have a solid basis for this assessment other than to feel there are forces at work that steer our boats when we aren't. More on this later too.

Speaking of steering our boats, while I never got to fly a jet—one of my yet unfulfilled dreams—I did have a fairly unique experience while in Navy Dive School at Panama City (you may recall that I was in the Army with Special Forces then). We all went out to sea to drop divers into the ocean to walk on the bottom as part of the training with surface-supplied air hoses wearing dive suits and helmets with little windows allowing a view of the ocean at depth.

On the way back to port, the Captain of this 300-foot vessel invited me to the bridge and asked me if I wanted to drive. You can imagine my response. So there I was at the helm of this ship behind this big wheel, holding my course, heading us back to port—no land in view—with a pod of dolphins leading our ship home. While this was an unusual experience and very exciting, anyone of you could have done it too. I asked the skipper if I could park it when we made it back to the dock, but this request was denied. I can't imagine why.

I had to add one more story since it illustrates the extraordinary showing up in our lives when unexpected. So let's just say at some point in time we discover we are on a path—not good, not bad—just a path. This path may be to family life, a chosen type of work, an art or craft, school or higher education, a career, a profession, an exploration of the world or of cultures around the world.

This path could even be we are headed to jail for some reason, very unlikely a chosen one, and certainly not seen as an optimal path, but one in which we can learn and grow from, or not.

I used the expression *very unlikely a chosen path* since I know from personal experience that some inmates when released, commit a crime just to get back in again feeling more comfortable there than in the outside world—this as revealed to me by an SF soldier in my unit describing his brother who was in prison, got out, then *had to get back in again* so committed another crime.

See this as just another path, another set of experiences. If we are thrust onto a path, we can consider changing it—except in jail, fewer options there—but they do exist there too, really—and we may just have to wait until we get out to make our mark in the world. But you see my point.

No path is wasted. It is just an experience to love, hate, or be somewhere in between. I'll put my money on loving your path as it seems to be a better choice and a better experience. Ask the ones who love their path. Even they will admit to some hardships along the way. That's life.

So give this careful consideration as you choose what you want to do in your life. And there are always opportunities to change your mind. Many may feel they are trapped. They aren't. That's just a story they've made up about themselves. Not everyone will agree but that's okay.

How do you pick a path? Well, I talk to my patients all the time these days about picking a path to feel better, get over an illness, change course, etc. I simply suggest they ask themselves and then come up with an answer right away.

Alternatively, they can consider, say five things, and write them down, quickly. The number doesn't matter—it's just a framework, a starting point—not too much thought though. Thinking gets in the way sometimes. Just be spontaneous. And be playful with this exercise, not serious. Usually better results. Rely on your intuition. If you don't think you have any intuition, just develop it and practice. This subject of Intuition is worth a later chapter in this book. If you don't think you have any intuition, just imagine it. By the way, that's another chapter in this book— Imagination.

Right now, I'm just glad you picked a path to read this book. You won't recognize yourself by the end of it, but you may recognize your SELF. And you may find you have more path choices at the end of it. Remember my comments in the Introduction about having a Bilbo Baggins Adventure. Well, this is one of them. Enjoy it, embrace it. Don't dread it or fear it or worry about it. Remember the movie, Bridge of Spies, when Tom Hanks (as a lawyer defending a Soviet spy in the US) asked the spy, "Aren't you worried?" The spy, asked, "Would it help?"

Chapter 3
KEEPING IT SIMPLE

You heard me mention this earlier. I like simple. It speaks of effortless ease. Simple is not a philosophy. It is a quality. There is no formula for *simple*. It is for each of us to figure out what constitutes *simple* in our life and choose to act on it, live it to the best of our ability, or not.

If we choose to learn from our ancestors, or from those who walked upon the earth a long time ago, or choose to learn from the words of the masters, the seers, the rishis, the wise ones, or perhaps even from our own inner guidance—call it intuition, imagination, source, whatever you like—then pay attention and listen more mindfully. You see I believe it is all connected. We are all in touch with everything there is to know in every moment, but most of us are not aware of this. This idea is not original with me either. A lot of people much smarter and wiser than me have shared this notion with the world. You do not need to buy into it, but perhaps consider it. Remember, do not trust a word of what I say—and this is not the last time I will say this.

I will say that as part of our SELF discovery, exploration and inquiry may be part of it. You can put forth effort into this, but you don't need to. And practice, there will be lots of opportunity to practice as we uncover mystery upon mystery. Sounds exciting, doesn't it? . . . I'm writing it and it sounds very exciting to me too!

So where do we begin with introducing *simple* into our lives? I don't know for you but for me I first had to get comfortable with the

KISS principle. It used to refer to the phrase, *keep it simple, stupid*, but later I read someone's interpretation of it as *keep it simple, smarty*. This to me implied it is smart to keep something simple. I liked that. Did I mention that I like simple too? :)

How do we distinguish simple from not simple, from complicated, complex? Just look into your life. I have had much complicated and complex in my life. Even the prefix *com-* means it comes with something, more stuff perhaps! I now easily can see where I sabotaged myself, not intentionally, just noticing, looking back. That's the beauty of hindsight. The trick is catching hindsight before it happens. That's why it's called foresight. We can get good at this with practice, but first we need to develop . . . that's right . . . awareness! You see how easy this is? You got that right away.

Simple belongs in the hands of the beholder, for each of us to determine for ourselves. You see, my simple is not your simple and vice versa. We each have our own version of it. The important thing perhaps is that we recognize simple may be a more luminous and less cluttered path. It may not be either, but I offer it is at least worth a try. There is evidence that this is true. Just ask anyone who has discovered this in their own lives. As Tony Robbins once said in a course that included a Fire Walk that I did with him years ago, "Success leaves clues."

I am not saying that *busy* does not occur in our lives. It does. It is how we respond to busy that affects us, either adversely or beneficially, or somewhere in between.

Most of us have our *to do* lists—things we must do no matter what. Most of us work to make an income to pay our bills, to feed our families, to take care of and provide for our children or our aging parents, to pursue our dreams. Many of us must pay taxes, household bills, rent or mortgages, things we feel are necessary in our sphere of life in our communities.

The question I will pose to you, is this working for you or is it slowly suffocating you, or maybe burying you in an avalanche? If it is working for you and you are content with your life and feel peace and calm, then skip to the next chapter. If you are like most of us, we can do with a little more *simple* and *calm* in our lives. It is also part of achieving good health and vitality. Do you want any of that?

I will only briefly mention some ways to achieve simple and calm. These are all time tested and proven to be effective. If you try them and they don't work, feel free to discover your own ways. Remember we are all unique beings and possess the gifts of imagination and creativity toward fulfilling our dreams if we choose to awaken to this path. Remember to explore your intuition too.

Most of us have heard of the value of finding stillness, meditation, being in and around Nature, experiencing timelessness, loving unconditionally (a biggy!), and finding joy within ourselves regardless of what is happening in our external world (another biggy!). There is also Yoga—yoking the mind and body, causing the cessation of mind chatter (Yogas chitti vritti narodaha, remember?), and any form of exercise done mindfully. Many of us do exercise without regard for our bodies— we punish ourselves in the name of getting fit. Remember to always honor your temple, the one we were gifted coming into this life and the one we will leave behind when we depart.

Just for the fun of it, come up with a list of your own ways of finding simple and calm in your lives. Do you like to sing, dance, play an instrument, make music, write, paint, sculpt, do art of any kind? Remember doing your own life is a form of art (refer to the Introduction of this book). So be creative and see what shows up for you. Do your own version of whatever brings you simple, peace, calm, and whatever you wish to bring more of into your lives.

This chapter will be short, in keeping with my intention of keeping it simple. This is now up to you to decide if simple is a smart direction for your life—whatever your path. If you decide it is, then start looking at your life in great detail over the years and see where you let complex and complicated and too busy and too distracted, etc. etc. enter into it. No guilt or feel bad if you see it but learn from what life has offered up to you to help you see more clearly. If nothing comes up that is okay. Perhaps in time something will show up. There is no wrong way here, only learning experiences and opportunities to grow, become more aware, and evolve—also, our experiences and opportunities to grow are unique to each and every one of us.

That's it for this chapter. Simple, wasn't it?

Chapter 4
QUALITIES OF LIFE AND LIVING

Perhaps the first important question to ask ourselves is, are we living? . . . Not like alive and breathing, walking, and talking, but truly living? Does anyone see the distinction? I didn't either for a long time. I think anything this good to recognize and acknowledge should be embraced as early as possible. Why wait for this quality called truly living, truly experiencing life at a higher more joyful, more heart- centered way, if perhaps it is available to all of us now?

I know many will note that we need to pay our dues, our karmic debt, suffer life's difficulties, earn our stripes, before we can graduate to a higher plane of reality, a higher consciousness, an awakening to the unseen world that we are all part of. Or do we?

I have been on this planet for a few years—this time. I'm not sure that there are any shortcuts to awakening and experiencing the good life now, but I'm willing to explore the possibility and share anything I find of value. In this light, be prepared for what I say. This is from my experience and my journey and may not work for you. I also said I would not be saying anything within the covers of this book if I did not find it of value to you. It is up to you to determine the truth of it or not for yourself. It just takes an open mind. An open heart may help too.

On the subject of *open heart*, what do you think this expression means? You see, I believe strongly that how life shows up to us is a reflection of how we show up to ourselves (and to others). Some of us, maybe most of us, associate the heart with something more than an organ that pumps blood around our bodies to oxygenate our cells and sustain our lives. The heart is also a symbolic representation of love for a number of us, would you agree? Why not the foot, or the head, or any other part of the body? No, the heart won those honors for some reason, and it has stuck for millennia. From the wisdom of Ayurveda, the mind is considered to be in the heart, not the head.

So when I use the phrase, open heart, it speaks to me of the opening of oneself to love, to love others, to love life, to love oneself, to love anything. Now there is the word, love, and there is the experience of love, two very different qualities depending upon our interpretation.

I am going to speak of the experience of love, the cosmic glue I mentioned earlier, the force that is everywhere, that is intelligent, and that connects all things with all other things. Just a thought to explore . . . and you know what I'm going to say . . . don't believe a word I say. Just explore what you feel about this quality. Perhaps explore your intuition. Perhaps ask your heart what it has to say, and then listen to its response.

I will suggest that those of us that embrace this quality of love in life for ourselves, experience a world with love in it. I will also suggest that those of us that consistently experience anger or hate or jealousy or envy or greed or resentment, or any combination of these qualities, see more of this in the world. Feel free to identify other qualities that you feel should be on this list too.

If we embrace kindness, compassion, understanding, sharing, love, joy, as part of who we are, then these qualities seem to show up in the world more for each of us. These thoughts are not new with me, but I will tell you I've experienced all of what I stated above as true for me, the good, the bad, and the ugly. I also have observed in the deeds, the actions, the experience of others, that this seems to play out too. I don't know for certain—just an idea to consider. And you can name more qualities that you wish to identify and manifest in the world as you wish—no limitations of the good stuff as you see them.

It can be stated even more simply. We either do things in life out of fear or we do them out of love. What we do out of fear is not done out of love. And what we do out of love has no basis in fear. There is a difference. Try it out for yourselves. And as an example, consider a mother afraid of water, jumping into water to save her child. If you look around you may note that far more of us act out of fear than out of love. Look honestly and deeply into your own life. What do you see?

I will suggest something really radical now. If you love yourself— read that as loving your SELF unconditionally—then you perhaps only see the world as loving, as a place of love. And if you are not acting out of fear, if you see that there is nothing to fear, you do not see the world as something to be feared, as a fearful place to live. That is not to say that there are not dark and dangerous things in the world.

It is to say if you don't fear them, you may not attract them to you. You may have heard the expression that we attract to ourselves that which we fear most. To sum up this notion, the universe rearranges itself to reflect back to us that which we see, that which we are, that which we need to learn in order to evolve.

I know this might take a stretch of your imagination, your belief system, maybe challenges your previous down payment on buying into consensual reality, but just consider it. Remember, nothing has happened to you. You are just reading words and considering ideas.

You may also consider I have your best interests at heart. I have nothing to sell you, to convince you of, to market, other than perhaps the opportunity to break free of pre-existing bonds that you may never have considered existed, in order to free yourself for an extraordinary life. I would also ask you to consider making yourself far more valuable than you thought you were before. Once considered, you may never look back again, being too busy discovering a new you and re-inventing your Self along the lines of your dreams.

I must confess to an ulterior motive in writing this book and sharing these words with you, and the motive is, I desire your life to be everything you ever dreamed it to be, whatever you want it to be—amazing, extraordinary, health-filled, vital, unimaginably wonderful, joyful, adventurous, fun, you name it! That's it. That's my confession. And there is a request hidden within this motive, that once realized, once experienced, that you pass it on, pay it forward, to anyone you choose.

Now, if you just stay with me for the following chapters, we will look together at how we may construct this life, this very unique and personal dream, this life of living fully, not just being alive. I'm still excited! How about you?

Chapter 5
LIVING FULLY NOW OR LATER

This is not Life 101. This is the Advanced Course which you did not know you were signing up for when you picked up this book. My intention is that you get your life out of this book, not like you don't already have one, but that perhaps you'll hardly recognize the one into which you are evolving, or will barely recognize the one you left behind, will hardly be able to imagine that was you.

By the way, I have imposed the same standards on myself. I do not intend to recognize myself—the person I was—when this is complete. You may say we are on this journey together and believe me it is every bit of a Bilbo Baggins Adventure that I referred to in the Introduction. My children will be happy to see I included this notion of outrageous adventure and risk-taking in this book.

Oh, and for those readers who identify themselves as non-risk takers, as wall flowers, as 'thanks-but-I'd-rather-not-participate' people, stay tuned. You will be amazed at what you will discover within your Selves as the seeds we are planting take root and you allow them to grow and sprout and seek sunlight with effortless ease.

This work may take some courage, to confront some things you are not currently confronting. But I will wager that once you start sensing what lies ahead for your life, what may be a transformation of your life, a transcendence into another way of being, that say possibly, just maybe, 100% of you will take this on and rise to the occasion. Your life is in fact a celebration, something to be toasted to, something to be artfully designed with more than a significant amount of imagination—just like the title of this book.

I want to admit, that there is much of my life that was not comfortable, that there has been much uncertainty, much insecurity, and much not knowing, going on. I also want to say that I have much more fully moved into living in the NOW moment, not worrying about tomorrow, or regretting what happened yesterday. This is a very liberating experience. You may have heard this before, from the Power of NOW (Eckhart Tolle), and from many other authors. Because I have discovered the wisdom of uncertainty, the freedom in allowing myself to feel insecure, my life unpredictable, my not knowing how something is going to turn out, I have discovered my SELF—I have discovered Me in a much different light, in a much different world.

At first, due to life events and circumstances, I sat with a lot of sadness, pain, loneliness, heartache, over the course my life had taken. Sounds dramatic, doesn't it? I will elaborate on these events later in this book to illustrate a few points common to us humans. Yet each one of these emotions, and all my experiences (the good, the bad, and the ugly) served as my teachers, as blessings in disguise, eventually casting a light onto the path that I was to take, illuminating my way even in the darkness (that sounds pretty dramatic too, but it's actually pretty true).

For me to see this path, I had to look for it. I had to involve myself in my own life. I had to be willing to experience the dark night of the soul to walk more fully into the light. This appears to be a common experience for humans, perhaps all of us, the experiencing of the dark night of the soul.

Anyway, I decided I had to be with it, to embrace the pain and difficult emotions at my core, at my heart's center, and not choose to escape via alcohol, drugs, pharmaceuticals, denial, jumping off a building, whatever we humans come up with to avoid facing our demons. In other words, I went inside to look deeper. I did not go to a therapist but briefly. Therapy is not a bad choice. It just wasn't my choice.

So to get back to Living Fully Now or Later It becomes just a matter of saying yes to it, to choosing now rather than later, to be willing to look at any and all obstacles in our way to becoming all that we desire to become, to letting go of all that which no longer serves us anymore and walking away from it whether we are 20 or 90, or even younger or older. I am doing this now as I write. We are in this experience together.

This journey of being with and letting go can be done alone. To have close friends or a committed listener or a loved one in our life who really cares about us, helps. I will also suggest that as we learn to tap into the intelligent universe all around us, there is no end to the support we can perceive and receive—a good time to practice your imagination and intuition. The unseen world exists, and is far more real than the illusory world of manifestation that we live in. More on this later, but those of you who have already experienced this know what I'm referring to.

It now becomes clear that we should all decide what living fully looks like to each of us. What is your version of living life fully, of living outside the 9 dots, of choosing a life without boundaries or limitations, of living life artfully with great imagination?

I know there are laws and rules and things that we feel confine us or restrict us, but these are all manmade constructs and illusion. There are Laws of Nature and Laws of Spirit that are worth considering and embracing but they exist in a very different way than the rules and laws and norms of any society.

You see we live with and within Nature. We are Nature. And we are Spirit. Spirit is us. Therefore, embracing and paying attention to these so-called laws of Nature and Spirit may be a good idea. Think of it like the sun shines everyday even if it is a cloudy day. The sun just is. It is its Nature to shine, to warm, to illuminate our world. And this phenomenon may exist on other worlds with suns (stars) too. In fact, I'll take a chance and assert that it does in a way unique to that star system within that galaxy.

Of course, if you break a law in any society, there will be consequences, so out of your own self-interest and self-preservation, be mindful to not breaking any laws if you don't want to risk accumulating bad karma, go to prison, or worse, depending upon the society in which you live. There are exceptions here too but mostly in a civilized world this boils down to respecting others and their boundaries. We must also consider what it means to show up as civilized.

So just for the fun of it, take a moment to write down on one page—or two at the most for now—what your life would look like if you were living fully. Be bold! Be imaginative! Most importantly, be the most amazing you that you can design without reservation! There is no room here for what anyone else may think, for consensual reality. Pretend for a moment that you are the only human being in the world and that you can do anything you want, be anything you want to be. What shows up for you? Then bring the people back in since we live in community.

And what we will invent together in the rest of these pages is a way to manifest that reality of living fully for each of us. We know that as many of us that are walking the planet right now are the number of ways to live fully that will surface. We are all unique. Let's live as if this is so, because it is.

Chapter 6
REINVENTING OURSELVES

Now that most of us—maybe all of us—have decided we would like to be living life fully right now, we may be wondering how we get there from where we are. Remember, this is the Advanced Course on living life, and I will be talking to you with great respect and love and honoring the human beings we are—each of us possessing unlimited possibilities and a power to create extraordinary things.

I mentioned earlier that we each are so much more than we think we are. Why I am writing this book is because I was fortunate enough to experience certain things in my life that I thought were genuinely important to pass on—and this because I was fortunate enough to be blessed with the experience of caring about Mother Earth and all her beings. And all this seems to spill out of my interest in exploring what creates great health and vitality and wellbeing for each and every one of us. You see, it's all connected. We are all connected. I may mention this again.

Some of us may not feel we are living fully in this moment. Perhaps most of us don't feel that way. I didn't either for the longest time. I still don't sometimes. But I got my eyes on the prize, this elusive life of living my dream. And it is definitely manifesting little by little, sometimes in spirts, sometimes in big leaps. Before I was too busy to even notice where I was going or what I wanted to create for myself. That is changing. One way of getting here was learning to reinvent myself.

I'm speaking personally about me and my dream now. You have the same capacity to do this too. Just change the scenery for your own dream, to your images for the life you desire. Then jump into creating it. This all starts with a single thought and your intention to take that first step on your path to your new reality.

Part of reinventing ourselves includes looking at the story we have created for ourselves. We all have a story. Many of us aren't even aware we have a story. We just live it like we have no choice. But we do. There are stories that restrain and restrict us in life, imprison us. Many of us are not aware that we live in a cage with an unlocked door, and still feel we are locked in and unable to fly free. Some of us live in that cage and the door is visibly open and we are still afraid to fly free of it.

I know people like this. I've been one. I'm not one anymore—part of the reinvention process.

There are also powerful stories in life—many of them. We can choose one of these. We may already have chosen one or are living a really good story worth sharing. Stories have been told for ages with amazing effects on the listeners. Then too, many stories are not experienced as so empowering or enlightening. The listener gets to decide, not the storyteller. However, the storyteller may be very aware of how powerful her or his story is, and that's why they tell it. The role of the storyteller is another story. We'll get back to this later. For now, I just want to encourage all of us to come up with good stories about ourselves and our lives that are worth sharing with our families, our friends, our communities.

Keep in mind that we have all told stories, and heard stories, that have us go unconscious, fall asleep, mutter, "Oh God, not that one again!" So, pick a different story that enrolls your listener. Stories help when they get someone excited about their own life. It's kind of like sorting through the junk mail—if it's junk mail, it goes right into the trash. No sharing. Keep that in mind. Your Higher Self may be of value here. Get familiar with checking in with it. Get used to quieting down your Monkey Mind also, which is always willing to share an opinion but often of little value. You'll soon discover the difference if you haven't already.

Just for the fun of it—you may notice I say, "just for the fun of it" occasionally. This is natural for me, and I also want you to start thinking about generating this quality more in your life, this quality called FUN. Be playful, imaginative, creative, have fun! So, just for the fun of it, write down your story right now, any story, perhaps one you tell often about yourself, about your life, your joys or woes. Then read it. Do you like it? Do others like it? If you don't like it, rewrite it. Yes, right now! Rewrite your new story in a way that it excites you and excites others. Of course, make it up! I don't want you to write a story about your life—made up or real— that you don't like. Write it like you are preparing to live it so make it good.

By the way, that is exactly what I did in my life. I made up this crazy, wonderful, fantastic story that got me so excited I practically jumped out of my skin! Actually, I did jump out of my skin. In fact, I jumped way beyond my body to come up with what I imagined. Then I set about living it, my intention now to manifest every bit of it in my life.

I'm not there yet, but I'm getting glimpses and experiences that I'm on the right path. I've had disappointments, setbacks, breakdowns, breakups, joy vanishing at times, only to return again. Now I never give up. Spirit assures me that perseverance is important in the pursuit of our dreams. You might say that I have seen the light. By the time this book is finished I'll have more to tell you. But meanwhile I am living life in a very fulfilling way—call it living life fully NOW, not later! And this moment called NOW is the only moment we are truly alive.

This was another simple chapter, was it not? Does anyone not see how easy it is to write up a story that represents the dream you would like to manifest in your life? Manifesting this dream is another matter, and the map, the terrain, the compass, and the navigator, and the consciousness and intelligence behind all these items, will be further discussed on the following pages. Is there anyone who does not want to continue this journey with me at this point?

If anyone responded No to that last question, please read the next chapter, because perhaps I have failed to get you excited about your own life up to this point. The next chapter will fix this. Thanking you in advance for staying with me.

Chapter 7
MANIFESTATION—CREATING THE LIFE YOU ONLY DREAMED OF UNTIL NOW

I know I warned you that this was the Advanced Course, and not Life 101. I also warned you not to believe a word of what I say since I'm making this all up. That said, I want to invite you to play with me in this increasingly outrageous journey we are taking together toward the manufacture of—read that as toward the manifestation of—the life you desire, no holds barred. I said manufacture because we are also building something together. Manufacture captures the essence of constructing something.

I also think of the word manifestation in magician's terms, like making a rabbit appear out of a magician's hat, or a dove out of his or her coat sleeve. I will introduce the notion that we are perhaps all magician's becoming—we are all wizards-in-training, wizards in the making of magic. Don't fall asleep or duck out yet. I really am a grounded human being, and if referring to the stripes I have earned is important to you, please do so. They used to be my roles and a variety of robes I used to wear in a society that places great importance on such things.

However, as part of my Shamanic training I have learned the importance of discarding those roles and robes, preferring to show up naked in life—as the authentic me doing the rest of my journey. That is not to say that my achievements and accomplishments in life were not important to me at the time. They were. They still are in a detached sort of way. They were part of my journey and still serve a purpose. It's just that they aren't me anymore. They served my ego until I decided my ego would be subservient to the Spirit which inhabits this human form.

We all have egos. We could just allow either our lives to be ruled by our egos or be connected to Spirit in a deep and all-abiding way, the ego becoming VP, second-in- command, an XO (executive officer), whatever. The ego goes nowhere. The ego is important to us humans. It just doesn't command the ship anymore. You can also think of it as a First Mate if you will, and Spirit as the Skipper.

You may notice that I use a lot of nautical terms—that's because I am a sailor and I love the sea. You will see lots of references to sailing our ships, calm waters or turbulent seas, charting our course—I have been there and have lots of fond memories from the ocean, and from being on it, in it, or under it (I also dive as I mentioned—great world down there, a whole other different world actually).

And if you really want to jump to the head of the class in this Advanced Course of Life, consider that we are the sea too. This is an advanced notion that I am of course making up, but also, I did not originate this idea either. It has been around for a long time and part of ancient wisdom and ancient teachings long before the written word. This of course can be verified with a little research.

Some of you may have heard it expressed that we are all part of the One, that we are all ONE. This is a tough one to wrap our heads around. But just try this on for a while and see how it sets with you. You don't need to buy into it, but it does tie in with the notion that we are all connected to everything and that everything is connected to everything else.

I know that I mentioned this earlier. Just let it marinate with you as we settle into the rest of this journey together. By the way, I totally accept this. It is not only useful but totally works in my life. There may be some examples of this later. And I'm pretty sure that some of you have some great examples in your own lives to share on this experience of Oneness too.

I mentioned this notion of Oneness at this time because the topic of this chapter is Manifestation. You see, if you intend to manifest something in your life, something that now seems improbable, or even impossible, it helps to have help. It helps to have guidance in discovering how to create something you dream about. Now you can have a Guru, a Saint, a Shaman, a Wizard, in your life to ask the tough questions of, but they will likely refer you back to yourself—more accurately to your Self.

You see, I believe the Self has all the answers. For this conversation in this Advanced Course, I see Self Equals Spirit—the SELF, or Higher Self, or big S, is one and the same as Spirit, Source, all that is, whatever you want to name it. Remember, it is in the knowing and not the label. Call your experience of the One or of Source anything you want to call it, if you can even accept it and believe it in the first place.

I practice this with my patients too. When I ask them what they think brought on the condition that they are consulting me about, most will say (if they truly don't have an idea), "I don't know." To which I then say, "what if you did know, what would you say?" A surprising number will answer right away and are pretty accurate and right on target. The rest of the story can be teased out with a little more inquiry.

For those who can't really get to it, I say, "just make something up, anything." And most will comply. We get to it right away. They get to see that they had the answer all along and I was just useful in perhaps facilitating it and extracting it. This too gets better with practice. My patients are just as important in developing this as I am in eliciting it. We do this together.

Since we are on the theme of Manifestation, I will share a story with you. It is one of my own stories. It is actually about this book I am writing.

For the longest time I have dreamed about writing a book. I even shared with you how this title came about—in a dream I had. It took years for me to begin it—for lots of reasons that I made up why 'not now, too busy' was the answer. Until this past year when I took it on as something I seriously wanted to do. But I had help.

Several years ago, when I experienced my life as not turning out, despite all the outward appearances that I was very successful in the usual way we tend to measure success—I had a good education, a good chosen profession, a successful career in the military with Special Forces (many of whom I experienced as my brothers), a great family blessed with wonderful children, all now adults. However, I had an unsuccessful marriage that ended in divorce with the mother of my children despite putting my heart and soul into keeping it viable, not to mention healthy and happy and vital.

That marriage was followed by another marriage that also failed after a nine-year relationship. And I was the guy who identified myself as totally about creating a happy, loving family life and being there for my children and my wife no matter what. I was committed to creating a happy loving thriving vibrant family life for the rest of this lifetime. It still didn't work.

This is when I decided I couldn't do it on my own. I decided to surrender to Spirit— that whatever my life was about wasn't working and I needed help. This idea of surrender isn't new either. I had heard about it, read about it, knew of people who surrendered their life to God, or Spirit, or some higher Being or Reality or Cause. This was just an idea to me then, something I knew about but not yet a knowing for me. But it did get me started on the rest of my life and what I will describe as miracles becoming commonplace in my life.

I also had to accept that if I were truly surrendering to Spirit, that Spirit could do with me whatever Spirit chose, for Spirit's purpose in the World. This meant that maybe my life would be put to some really good purpose and perhaps get much better than I was currently experiencing it. It also meant that Spirit may decide that I was to leave this world for the next—that is, that I would die. Perhaps too, Spirit may decide that I should take on serious disease or disability, or some tragedy, to make some kind of useful statement to humanity. I didn't know. But I did know that I was taking on some kind of risk that anything may show up.

For many years I have lived as honoring my word, felt that I was only as good as my word, and if I didn't honor my word as myself that I was dishonest and out of integrity. I took this very seriously and it became who I was in life. I wanted to be as authentic as possible. I also wanted to be a good role model in my children's eyes. So this is how I showed up for Spirit. I didn't always live this way. Before my children I was a different human being. That story will be for later, if not in this book, then the next one. It will get told eventually.

Suffice it to say, I underwent significant transformation. I am still undergoing significant transformation but now from a more conscious and awakened state. Even though living as my word and living in integrity are firmly in place, the path does not necessarily become easier, and perhaps it becomes more difficult, or at least perceived as more difficult—until we begin to perceive it as easier.

It was out of this surrender that help appeared, help from the unseen world as I identify it—help from the world of Spirit. I will develop this with all of you in this Advanced Course as this book unfolds, but for now I will just tell the rest of this story of how this book came to be a reality, a manifestation of a dream.

It may be important for you to know that I have been writing poetry for some years now. I soon realized that I was not writing my poetry. I wasn't plagiarizing it. I was just allowing it to be written through me. Sometimes I could barely write fast enough to keep up with the words coming through me. Then I would read it and think, "Damn, that's good! I didn't write that!!" Some poems would write themselves without any editing needed. I am sure I will include some of my poetry in this book before it is done.

But by now you are all getting some insight as to where I am going with this. This book was just an expansion of what I was experiencing with my poetry. So, my confession to you is that I am not writing this book, I am just allowing it to be written through me. I am just allowing Spirit to tell a story through me that Spirit needs to tell, and I've agreed to be part of it.

And there's nothing special about me. I'm not a chosen one, just another human being that said yes to something bigger than myself. I just agreed to be part of the process and not take ownership of the process, that is to say, no ego involved here, just appreciation and gratitude for being able to show up as something bigger than me that may make a difference.

There is another clue here. I have written all I have written so far as is. This is all first draft stuff, and it is mostly unfolding like a final draft finished book. I suspect that by the time this goes to press it will look different, but I also feel that if this is exactly what shows up in the bookstore, or Amazon, or wherever new books show up these days, I am satisfied that Spirit said it best and exactly as it was to be stated. An editor or a publisher may decide differently but I trust that what is being told is just perfect as it is. This is another miracle in my life.

I will just say now that I told this story because it perfectly illustrates the manifestation of a dream, the very subject of this chapter. I have manifested other dreams this same way too—by enrolling the help of Spirit, of something beyond me and yet part of me, to help with the creation of something from the world of the unmanifest bringing it into the world of the manifest. I'm working on a really big one right now that is not a book. I hope that it becomes manifest before this book is complete, and if it is you can be sure I will mention it within the covers of this book. And I will leave this chapter intact so you will know that I was headed toward something big but not yet present in my life. The mystery, the uncertainty . . . drumroll please!

And as a heads up, I will eventually ask all of you participating in this Advanced Course with me to share your stories of dream manifestation with me. And if I have your permission, I will share some of your stories in a future book. Names add to the authenticity of the stories, and to the spice of acknowledging your life too, but if you wish to remain anonymous you may. Sounds exciting, doesn't it? And I will definitely be happy to add more of my stories to what we are creating together.

You see, I believe this is a direction that we humans are all headed—in the direction of dreaming our world into existence, into a world we wish to create for our children's children.

This is one of the things the Q'ero, the Shamans of the High Andes, are doing. The Andean Shamans are dreaming our world into existence for all of us—not a world based on the desires of the ego, not a world of taking advantage of others, or making a profit without sharing the wealth, but a world that is for the greater good of all humanity, for Mother Earth and all her beings. This is something that can perhaps get some of us out of bed in the morning and launched into an amazing day, launched into an amazing life, launched into a future that we can only dream about—or perhaps create with the help of Spirit.

So now you may have a formula for success for manifesting your dreams. This works. And you know what is to follow now—don't believe a word of this. Try it first and see if you can prove it in your life. If you can't, keep looking. You will find a way. Spirit assures me of this. There will be other ideas offered later that will assist in unlocking the doors of this mystery. Stay tuned.

But more important for this moment, as I inquired at the end of Chapter Six, how many of you have decided to bail on what we have begun together here? Have I succeeded in getting you excited about the possibilities of your own life, about your dreams not yet manifest, but to be? Have I enrolled you in continuing the rest of this journey together towards the creation of an amazing and extraordinary and miraculous life? . . . YOURS!

Chapter 8
PURIFYING MUDDY WATERS, SEEING BEYOND THE MIST

I believe that part of our journey—maybe the whole journey itself—is to arrive at clarity, to become enlightened beings, to evolve into pure Spirit. Just my notion. You don't need to subscribe to it. But it may be useful as you find your way on your own path. There are others who have felt this way too. The great masters I referred to earlier spoke of this, and many others since.

The next thing we will explore together is how do we get the mud to settle in the water we live in to become pure, or the mist to disappear, so we can see clearly. Pick any metaphor you like—the point is we are heading toward seeing clearly whatever lies before us, all around us, behind us, beneath us, above us, and within us. There are some shortcuts, some effortless ease ways to this seeing, yet some of us may be destined to doing it the hard way until we don't anymore. I've been there so I can speak to this. This is why I want to introduce some thoughts on making this easier for us, a quicker path to living life fully now.

First, there are clues everywhere. If you've missed them, perhaps it's only because you haven't been looking for them, or maybe too busy with your cell phone, or the TV, or gossip, or your own mind chatter, or the myriad distractions we humans fabricate that we have been calling living life or important but isn't really. We are kept pretty busy living someone else's idea of life. But it's not our life. We must discover what is our life about—more accurately, ask your Self, "WHAT IS MY LIFE ABOUT?" This was suggested in earlier chapters. This chapter is about refining our ideas and our vision of our selves. This chapter is about arriving at more clarity.

In keeping with my intention of keeping our work together simple and useful and understandable, I will suggest some things I have personally found helpful. Some of these things took me most of my life to arrive at, so if I can facilitate your path to discovery to make your life easier, I will. And there's always the hard way if you prefer that. And just in case you forgot, have some fun with this. They are just a bunch of words and ideas that I'm offering. It's up to you to bring them to life. Play with this!

I will mention a bunch of things that can be very helpful in seeing more clearly the life you are living—and once seen, your path may open up for you and become more illuminated. I have stated a number of these notions earlier, notions that finding stillness, meditation, Yoga, calming the monkey mind, being in and with Nature, are pathways to the divine, to the essence of your being.

I also mentioned qualities that bring you greater joy and the experience of love in your life, and other qualities that get in the way, qualities that if chosen (like anger, hatred, resentment, jealousy, etc.) have you experience your world reflecting those qualities back at you. So simply drop those qualities that don't serve you, that reflect the world back to you in an undesirable or unpleasant way. This takes some practice but is absolutely doable. Refer to the earlier chapters if you forgot these qualities. I will confess that I have reread some books that I found particularly good, six, seven, eight times and maybe even more. Can't get too much of a good thing sometimes. And I too appreciate the reminders.

It is important to tell the truth, I believe, to honor our word, to live as our word. Practicing loving kindness for all beings is good. Bringing compassion and understanding to all things in life works well too. While none of us may be perfect at living these qualities all the time, just being mindful that they exist, helps remind us and illuminates our path as we assist in illuminating the paths of others. Treat others as you wish to be treated—some of you have heard this before.

As I began to walk the path of a Shaman, participated in the Shaman's Altar, studied the Four Directions of the Medicine Wheel, I came into deeper relationship with the qualities of a Shaman and my relationship with Pachamama—Mother Earth. I have been aware of my relationship with some of these qualities for a long time, and also with my relationship with Nature and Mother Earth. I have deepened.

I will share some of these shamanic qualities with you. They are taken from my notes during the medicine wheel of my Shaman's Altar taught by Shamans Shanon and Marv Hardwood. You may adopt them or not. I am sure that at least a few of you have already brought these into your life. Just imagine if we all did.

QUALITIES OF A SHAMAN

A shaman practices non-judgment
A shaman practices non-attachment
A shaman learns to not take him/herself seriously . . .
A shaman learns to laugh at him/herself
A shaman does not cast a shadow . . . that is;
A shaman does not project his or her stuff onto another
A shaman tells the truth
A shaman does not like to be controlled
A shaman is Self-referencing
A shaman walks on the earth with integrity and impeccability
A shaman's intention is everything
A shaman evaluates the consensual reality and then makes his/her mind up for him/herself
A shaman practices staying in balance, at staying in Ayni

While I will not guarantee that living your life along the principles and qualities stated above will transform your experience of life, I will say that there is maybe a 99.9% chance it will. Oh, what the heck, let's just round it off and say there is a 100% chance it will transform your life. Please let me know if this isn't true for you and I will include it in my next book. You must however agree to practice all of these in your life for at least six months. See what shows up after that.

I want to say a word about books. There are lots of authors that I have read, and I respect greatly what they bring to the world, and to our better understanding of ourselves and the life we live. I honor them. As such I will at times reference them within the pages of this book. I will include a number of them as a suggested reading list at the end of this book. I have also written up a one-page reading list for any of my patients who are interested. I title this page that I offer my patients, **Books to Grow By.**

I've mentioned that I like simple. Some works simply state things that I believe are important to arriving at clarity, at living life in a fully engaged, healthy, wholesome, loving, vital way, and simultaneously are easy to read. This appeals to my love of choosing effortless ease as we learn and grow and evolve. I see this as a path to becoming a good human being, and being a good human being is a path to living life fully in a healthy vital way.

One such book that falls into the category of short, easy to read, and read-more- than-once by me, is Deepak Chopra's book, *The Seven Spiritual Laws of Success*. Deepak signed my copy when I did a course with him at Kripalu in Stockbridge, MA, nestled in the Berkshires, so it has a personal touch of his energy in it beyond his written words. I like Deepak and I respect him and what he brings to our world. This book provides a blueprint for living life that embraces the notion that we are much more than we seem to be in our basic human forms. This is not the first time I encountered this, but Dr Chopra states it clearly and simply in identifying these spiritual laws. Deepak states that we are pure Spirit having an occasional human experience rather than humans having an occasional Spiritual experience. I agree.

These seven spiritual laws could have been written by a Shaman. A Shamanic path embraces Spirit—the words or phrases (the literal) may be different. The Four Directions of the Shaman's Altar are about the Literal, the Symbolic, the Mythic, and the Energetic (the Spiritual). These are the four domains in which the Shaman engages, but especially the mythic and energetic.

The Four Agreements by Don Miguel Ruiz is another short, easy to read, not so easy to practice, book that addresses four agreements we can make and bring to our lives with great benefit. I mentioned Don Miguel earlier in the introduction. This book is worth reading too.

Returning to Kripalu, which I often referred to as my home away from home when I lived in New Hampshire, is where I trained as a Yoga instructor, took a number of other courses, and where I did most of my course work in Ayurveda. Dr Vasant Lad was one of my teachers. For those of you who haven't heard of him, get to know him. He has written more than a few books, my textbooks on Ayurveda among them. Be sure to read something by Dr Lad. He is still practicing and teaching at the Himalayan Institute of Ayurvedic Medicine in Albuquerque, New Mexico, which he founded in 1971.

You may recall that I mentioned Ayurveda in my introduction to this book. The wisdom of Ayurveda has much to offer on one's path to health and healing. Ayurveda offers that self-healing happens when we get out of our own way and allow it to occur. We'll come back to this. Ayurveda is known as the oldest, continuously practiced, medical science in the world, and is said to have existed before the written word. It is also said by some that there was never a time that Ayurveda didn't exist.

Ayurveda introduces us to diet and lifestyle considerations that help us cleanse and detoxify our bodies as we regain balance and purify our systems. As we regain balance (move into Ayni as a Shaman would call it—coming into reciprocity and alignment with the Universe and Spirit), we heal.

You see, Ayurveda offers that many of us live in a virtual sea of toxicity by virtue of the quality of the air we breathe, the food we eat, the thoughts we have, and the myriad unhealthy experiences we encounter, all building up *Ama* (toxic residue) in our physical, mental, and emotional bodies. If this Ama is not cleared out, this accumulation of toxic residue will eventually produce disease states. Healthy experiences and detoxification can rid us of Ama.

This is a very different approach than Western Medicine and one worth studying for all its added wisdom and guidance. If Ayurvedic principles alone are followed, your life will be transformed. An Ayurvedic path will be revisited throughout this book. It would serve you to study something of Ayurveda on your own too—a rich science of life. Start with Dr Lad's work.

At the risk of becoming more complicated at this point, you can see the take home message here—*simply stated*—is to choose to live a good life, be a good human being. You know the difference. You know when you are not being a good human being. If you don't know the difference, don't worry about it—you've got eternity to figure it out.

Choose healthy wholesome foods most of the time—it may not be always since we are after all, human. Choose healthy company too. If not experienced as a healthy choice, be the change that you would like to see more of in the world. Always do your best and be mindful in all things.

Choose acting out of love over acting out of fear. Choose to show up loving, compassionate, kind, caring, and mindful of Mother Earth and *ALL* her beings from all her kingdoms—including plant, animal, mineral. Treat all other humans as you wish to be treated, irrespective of race, country of origin, religion, gender, age, color, creed, status in life, and as many other categories that you can think of. If you come up with another category, automatically include it.

This is just the beginning of purifying muddy waters, of seeing through the mist we inherited by becoming human. In the pages ahead you will deepen your exploration and experience of the life you are choosing to live now from an uncommon place for many humans. And then, after you begin to see more light, to grow, to become more aware, you know what follows . . . Pay it forward, pass it on to your fellow travelers. Be the stone you throw into the pond of life creating ripples that spread throughout the universe. This is the journey. This is a true Bilbo Baggins Adventure.

Chapter 9
SEEING CLEARLY WITH NEW VISION

What exactly does this mean? For you, I don't know. For me, I'm beginning to get an idea of it. To be able to peer into the unseen world and see takes a little practice and getting used to. You just utilize other senses of perception. Imagination and visualization become your eyes. Listening to the words of guidance from the unseen becomes your ears. Feeling with your heart, your gut, your sense of intuition, becomes your sense of touch. Has anything *ever touched your heart?* All just refinements of our usual senses at a different level but so much more expansive and enriched.

And there is power here. In ***Why Me? Harnessing the Healing Power of the Human Spirit***, a book co-authored by Patricia Norris, PhD, and Garrett Porter, Patricia Norris tells the story of Garrett Porter, a 9-year-old boy with a brain tumor. After surgery, radiation, and chemotherapy the tumor was still there and growing. In later working with Pat Norris, Garrett invented his own system to combat the tumor after the failure of these other modalities.

I use the term *combat* because that is exactly what Garrett chose to rid himself of this *dangerous asteroid invading his solar system,* his chosen imagery. His immune response cells became starfighters that would blast away at this asteroid every night under his command before sleep. One day he announced to his parents that the tumor was gone. All that remained was a tiny white pea-sized remnant of the tumor.

Garrett's parents didn't believe him. It took a subsequent fall down his stairs at home with resulting head trauma for his parents to take him to the hospital. His doctor was incredulous. A CT scan of his brain revealed no more tumor—only a pea-sized calcification where the tumor had been. Garrett went on to college later, his occasional use of aids and sometimes a wheelchair was due to the impact of his surgery, and chemotherapy and radiation therapy on his brain tissue, not his imagined visualizations that ultimately won the war against this *invading asteroid*, his brain tumor.

Garrett's story is just one story. You may call it a miracle. There are many such stories and accounts of miraculous recoveries and healings. Read some of them. They are definitely out there all over the world. They speak of great possibility for the human condition. They usually don't make the headlines. In fact, many are not even believed. Look into some for yourself. They speak so loudly about what may be available to us humans.

These stories are of much greater value (my opinion) than most front-page stories in the daily newspaper, where nearly every day a brutal death, or a kidnapping, or a disaster, or a tragedy of some kind, can be found, or perhaps the revelations of a Hollywood star's latest romance or breakup. We have chosen to call this news.

With all due respect to the journalists who have made this their chosen life work, I am not sure what our—we the people's—fascination is with this form of news that instills more fear of life than inspires healthy heart-centered action for the common good of humanity. The short answer is it sells papers, it is what we seem to want to read. And to be sure, these stories are about someone else's life in almost all cases. This is another version of consensual reality, someone's idea that this should be important to our life. But is it? You will have to decide for yourself.

There is an organization founded in 1984 called the Giraffe Heroes Project. It features stories about common ordinary everyday people around the world who have been willing to stick their necks out (hence

71

the name Giraffe Project) for the greater good of humanity in some area of life. It often involves taking risks, even risk of death in some cases. This organization is growing worldwide, yet it is not part of regular dinner table talk like the other news stories mentioned above. Why do you think this is?

I mentioned these two stories above to perhaps inspire you with what's possible as a human. Before Garrett healed himself of a brain tumor under the care of Patricia Norris, only fear and dread were in Garrett's future—at least from his parent's points of view. Nothing was working up until his starfighters took over the battle.

And the Giraffe Project was just an idea before it was created and eventually took off—that ordinary people do extraordinary things but never make the news. I was at a conference when the Giraffe Project founders first described its inception at this program. I have since mentioned the Giraffe Project over the years. It inspired me. And it inspired me the times I felt that I was sticking my neck out. And I have at times, like in writing this book. I am sure it goes against the consensual reality of some.

In fact, I believe that a good many of my colleagues in Western Medicine would find this a difficult read. A lot wouldn't though because healthcare is experiencing its own awakening. This could be due to the practitioners however I must also credit my patients with leading this awakening.

When my patients know I'm not just about to suggest another test or offer up another prescription of which they are doubtful, they are relieved. When they begin to understand that I embrace a holistic philosophy, that I integrate Eastern and Western philosophies of healing and the energetics behind them, that I embrace the roles of healthy nutrition and healthy lifestyle choices on our paths to regaining or maintaining good health, they begin to share their own amazing stories with me.

Some of my patients have mentioned all the natural foods or natural remedies they are already taking with beneficial effect. They also would sometimes admit that their previous healthcare providers would not listen to them, would in fact invalidate their experiences with complimentary or natural therapies.

In summary, to see clearly is a good thing, I believe. For those of us who think we don't, just give up that notion. It is right around the corner since this book caught your attention, and you are still reading. Most of us haven't seen clearly since we were newborns. I recall hearing many years ago that in the first few days, weeks, or months of life after we are born, we spend a lot of time hanging out with God. You can interchange Spirit or whatever higher power you feel comfortable with in the naming of it. Remember, it is in the knowing and not in the labeling.

This then seems to precede the humanization we all go through as we are exposed to the way others think we should live our lives. It seems we come into a world of fleeting clarity and clear vision, called pure being—which we are unable to describe to our human caretakers when only days or months old—then spend most of our lifetime in muddy water or mist until we find a way back to clarity and a new vision of our Selves. This book is about reacquainting you with your SELF. If it can come about sooner rather than later in our journeys, I think that is worthwhile. Why not?

This all may appear like that fruit hanging in the tree just above our reach but accessible with a little ingenuity and imagination. I think you are all up to it. I know I am, and if I am, I know you are too. Let's reach together, or maybe stand on one another's shoulders, or something similarly creative.

And once plucked from the branch above us, we can share it.

And remember, someone else's clarity is not your clarity. We are all unique. No consensual reality allowed in unless you have first evaluated it and can then embrace it as your own. There may exist similarities and things we hold in common that will assist each of us with clarifying our vision but be ever mindful of our unique nature and connection to Spirit. And trust this. Therein lies the journey before us, and it is up to each of us to find our way.

Chapter 10
SPIRIT IS IN COMMUNICATION WITH US ALL THE TIME

I believe this is true. Actually, I know this is true. You'll have to discover this for yourself before accepting it. We only need to refine our listening skills to hear this voice that is always there for us. As noted earlier, these thoughts, ideas, notions, experiences as shared, are for you to consider, engage with, experiment with, or simply walk past without looking further or exploring in your own life. I think there is value here, which is why I am mentioning it.

There were clues mentioned above in the preceding chapters to acquire more stillness, quiet, and calm in your life to perhaps enable you to *hear* better, or *see* better, to *feel* all the life going on around us which I suspect for many of us goes unnoticed . . . until we notice. This would describe me and my earlier experiences of not noticing. Then I began to notice. Then I began to notice more and more. Then my life began to change.

My mentor and teacher in my Shamanic training, Marv Harwood, who is a Shamanic Elder trained in Plains Native Shamanism (and whom I spoke of earlier), has this to say about how Spirit communicates with us in ever-increasing increments in an effort to catch our attention. *First it is heard as a soft whisper. Then if we aren't listening, a bit louder whisper, then more volume if still unheard. If we still fail to listen, maybe a tap on the shoulder, followed by a harder tap or a nudge to get our attention. If that still fails, Spirit wraps us "up the side of the head with a two by four!"*

I have needed the two by four more than once in my life to pay closer attention to what was unfolding in my life—to wake up! This eventually taught me to listen more closely to Spirit's subtle messages. In other words, we can learn the easy way or the hard way. Both eventually work. Which way would you rather learn? And remember, we are in no rush. We have eternity to work this out.

This story reminds me of earlier stories of Spirit. Maybe my first encounter to raise my awareness of something more out there, came when I was in high school. My father offered me a book to read **Beyond Human Knowledge** by Raynor C Johnson.

It was interesting and revealing and was my introduction to the world of the unseen. I don't even recall much about it anymore other than it made an impact on me, perhaps preparing me for more to come. It wasn't until later that it occurred to me that if this information was beyond human knowledge, how was I able to read it?

I also recall a course I did in Boston while I was training in Orthopaedic Surgery at the Tufts-New England Medical Center Hospital. Our course facilitator, Lenny, asked us at one point if we were interested in meeting our Spirit guides. We all agreed. He pointed out that we could have a guru or other master appear in our external physical lives to lead us into deeper awareness if we could arrange it. Lenny also said that we all had access to our own inner guides that we could meet if desired. This was to become for me the first of many meetings with my guide. I don't know about the other course participants. I do recall that only I and one other participant that weekend actually met our Spirit guides through the deeply relaxing guided meditation into which Lenny led us.

We were all lying comfortably on the floor as we were instructed to close our eyes, begin a relaxation process of all the muscles in our body and to clear out any thoughts that may be in the way of this relaxation. It was then suggested that we each choose a location—real or imaginary—that for each of us represented a beautiful and serene place for a meeting of this nature. Lenny also told us that our Spirit guide would have a message for us.

I chose a place from my imagination. It was a beautiful small pond with a waterfall spilling into it on the far side. I was sitting on the bank on ultra-green soft and fragrant grass. All senses were enrolled as I heard the sound of the falls, birds chirping, saw butterflies fluttering, noted the fragrance of flowers nearby, and felt the warmth of the day, the feel of the grass beneath me, and the excitement of anticipation. I was in shade from the leaves of the tree above me, but the sun was shining, and the sky was a beautiful blue. I wasn't just picturing this—I was there!

My guide appeared across from me. He (my guide was a he) appeared luminous but clearly in the form of a human, almost transparent but his features so easy to visualize. I greeted him. He returned the greeting not as a stranger but as a friend who has known me for a long time. He knew me and my name. I asked him his name. He told me it was Gaemu without hesitation.

There was little said between us, just savoring the experience of this first meeting at the side of the pond with a waterfall. I asked if he had a message for me. He did. He told me I was to *teach Love*. That was all. We said goodbye but with a clear knowing that we would meet again.

That was my experience while I was with Gaemu. The experience of the other course participants, and Lenny's of me, was much different. Lenny said I stopped breathing. That my eyes rolled back, even though I had closed them initially. My chest wasn't moving with breath for minutes. Then I began shaking all over. It took a long time to come back as he told me later. The rest of the class were seated in a circle around me just observing me. What was this?

And what Lenny alone saw, which he shared with me and the other participants, was that he saw a bright ray of light coming into me, that he saw me as encased within an eggshell, and that the shell cracked open and fell away from me. He referred to this light as the *Christ Light* and explained I had just undergone an initiation. As I mentioned above, my body began shaking uncontrollably at the time of this experience. I was unaware of this.

Gaemu and I did meet again. But it was not until days later, maybe even a week or two later, that I summoned the courage to chance a second meeting, perhaps doubting that Gaemu would even appear for me. He did, as soon as I ventured to that realm and to that same location by the pond with the waterfall. This time it was like meeting an old friend.

That was the second of many meetings with Gaemu over the years yet before me then. Whether meeting formally by the pond, or casually with just an awareness he was right over my shoulder, guiding me based solely upon my question or inquiry into my concern of the moment. He is there now as I sense his presence whenever I reach out.

Those of you who have met your Spirit guides know what I'm talking about. Many have. Those of you who haven't, another adventure lies in waiting for you as a doorway into a new world opens before you.

I have lots of stories. I will only share a few more in this chapter since it feels appropriate and serves to get the message of our connectedness with Spirit is total and available to each of us.

The first one I will share occurred right after my mother died in 1986. The next one while I was running in the forest years ago. And there are others, all pretty short but all serve to illustrate what is available to us.

I remember going to the cemetery the day after my Mom was laid to rest there. She had a traditional burial in a coffin. I remember wanting her to wear a crown of flowers around her head as she lay in her coffin at her viewing in the funeral home. I arranged for that, not the coffin but the crown of flowers. I also remember thinking after she died that she was now a butterfly emerging from her cocoon. I associated butterflies with flowers too.

As I was sitting by her graveside that next day, I asked her to give me a sign that she was okay. Minutes later, at the far corner of the cemetery but clearly visible, I noticed a butterfly—a monarch butterfly, orange with black and white markings fluttering toward where I was sitting. I kept watching it. I somehow knew what was going to happen, and it did. The butterfly flew toward me and alighted on my Mom's headstone.

I sat there in amazement contemplating what just happened. As I have learned we humans often require confirmation of extraordinary events. Such was true for me that day too.

My next request was, please Mom, just one more sign that you are okay. Minutes later a bunny appeared across the cemetery hoping in my direction. It stopped right in front of me near my Mom's headstone. That was extraordinary, but still not enough to convince me that my Mom was okay and answering me from the new world into which she just transcended.

I made another request for one more sign of assurance that she was okay. It was a dark and cloudy day with no holes of blue sky peeking through. The sun could be imagined behind dark clouds to the west but not seen shining. Then the clouds parted and allowed a sunray to shine down on the cemetery and mostly just illuminated the area where I was sitting. That convinced me. I never questioned her okayness after that. She indeed became a butterfly and emerged from her earthly cocoon.

Another story happened when I went for a run in a forest near my home in Keene, NH. I often ran on this woods trail near the Ashuelot River coursing through my town. On this particular run, I became aware of a presence of something, like a commotion or excitement but nothing was around me. I was alone in the woods, just me, the trail, the trees, the undergrowth, and the river. I actually heard voices, more in my head than with my ears. I stopped and paid closer attention. The trees were speaking to me, and they were aware that I was listening to them.

The exchange that followed was equally amazing and I have carried it with me every day of my life since then. The trees were so excited that a human was listening to them, that I was actually paying attention to them and what they were expressing, and that I understood them. We spoke to one another. Their excitement of the relationship that was being formed was not containable, for both of us—the trees and me. I have always appreciated the woods since early childhood and felt at home in them. I have had many long runs in the woods wherever I go, often choosing to intentionally get lost and running until I eventually found my way out.

Out of that first meeting, they expressed great joy in communicating with me consciously, knowing I heard them. I then asked, "What can I do for you?" They responded. I say *they* because I sensed there were many involved in this conversation even though it seemed like one voice which was clearly understood.

Their response was that I could help by raising we human's awareness of them, of their consciousness, acknowledging them and the work they consciously do in our world. I promised to do this, not knowing what this would look like. But there was no question that I would not honor their request.

How this showed up in my life was to eventually tell this story over and over again. I was also guided to create a course on our awareness of Nature—and Nature's awareness of us.

My military career has mostly been with Special Forces. We adapt to living off the land and learn to utilize whatever is available to us for food, shelter, camouflage, and survival. In essence we learn to live with Nature. In my case, our unit was trained in winter warfare given the theater of operations back then. We were trained in winter survival. Years later when the cold war ended and the perceived threat changed, we began training in desert warfare, a marked departure from training in the northern states of the US or in Europe during the winter months or training north of the Arctic circle in January at temperatures of 60 below zero.

I also had a civilian role in an organization called Mountain Medicine Education Inc. It was designed to offer programs to anyone interested in learning how to manage injuries or illness in a wilderness environment when help was not near at hand. We often offered this course in the White Mountains of New Hampshire in November. We also provided a course twice in the Himalayas, climbing to above Everest base camp (an altitude of nearly 19,000 feet) while teaching our program on High Altitude Medicine. Some of us developed symptoms of acute mountain sickness and became teaching examples while climbing or finding the need to descend.

It was for this organization that I designed *Nature and You, Success and Survival*. The rest of the course description read as follows: *Deepening Our Understanding of . . . Our Relationship With Nature . . . Our Awareness of Nature . . . Nature's Awareness of Us . . . And Discovering A Partnership For Life.* This program was also offered to Special Forces, as SF truly relies on Nature for survival at times. Some of my team members in SF were invited to participate, and eventually teach, in Mountain Medicine Education.

In deciding to design this course on *Nature and You* I began to research what we knew about interacting with the world of trees and the rest of the plant kingdom. What I discovered was remarkable and formed the foundation of the course I was to teach with Mountain Medicine.

I learned that there was indeed a lot of research into the world of plants, the experiments at the Findhorn Foundation in Scotland among them. It was clearly demonstrated by a series of experiments that plants have emotions, react to soothing or disturbing sounds, and even register alarm when a plant next to them is hacked to pieces. Much has been investigated since then. Read about it if interested. Just investigate the work done at the Findhorn Foundation for starters.

I started this class on Nature and You by asking from the front of the room, how many here have plants in their home? Hands went up. I then asked how many spoke to their plants? Some hands came down and a number remained up. I then asked how many get responses from their plants? All hands went down, and our class had begun. I related the studies at Findhorn among some others. I discussed what indigenous populations knew about Nature that most of us in modern society didn't know or forgot we knew.

I then explained we were all going to go outside to take part in an experiment. Each of us were to go out into Nature, which was all around us, identify something—A bush, a tree, a plant, a rock, a log, a leaf, or blade of grass, whatever we chose, and to form a relationship with it. They were asked to stay within the range of my voice. I then led them through a brief relaxation followed by a guided meditation which included a series of questions they were to pose to their chosen *object* in nature. The questions could be about anything, about their own life, about the object they chose to communicate with, or anything else. They were then asked not to filter the responses but to simply trust them and note them, however unusual the experience seemed.

When this was over, we all filed quietly back into the course room for sharing. What some revealed from this outdoor exercise in communication gave them great insights into their life and answers to their questions. Some shared that a new direction in life opened for them. For some this was a Bilbo Baggins Adventure.

Also in indigenous cultures of the world where humans live sustainably with Nature, whether in the Amazon, the high Andes of Peru, Native American cultures in the US and Canada, Africa, the Aborigines of Australia, and many other sites around the world, if a question was raised about the edibility of a plant or a cure for a disease or an ailment, a shaman, medicine man, or any individual so trained in communication with the plant kingdom, would just ask the plant for the answer, trusting the answer they would receive from the plant. This works. Research it if interested. Great stories to be uncovered.

There was also the time I was taking a course with the Theosophical Society in Boston. Our instructor was Mark Sullivan. He and his assistant were discussing things of an energetic and spiritual nature with our class. I remember lying in bed one night before our class the following day. I was thinking of a question to ask Mark, a deep question that I suspected he may know the answer to, and I knew that I didn't.

The next afternoon when I walked into the course room with that question on my mind and Mark standing in front of the class, he just shifted his gaze directly on me, looked into my eyes, smiled, and nodded yes. That was the answer I was looking for. He didn't even wait for me to ask it. It was uncanny how I knew in that moment that he knew, and that he answered me without speaking a word. I can still see it now as if he were standing in front of me at this moment.

There was also the time when my daughter, Paige, was in 6th grade in a rural country school in Westmoreland, NH, with fields and woods all around it. They had a field day one day, all students and the teacher filing outside for the experience. A bee flew into their midst at one point, the kids scattering, some screaming in fright. My daughter Paige knew about bees. I had introduced my children to many things of Nature when very young, including bees and how to talk to plants. Paige just stood still, extended her arm, her palm upright, welcoming the bee. The bee flew to her hand and alighted there briefly, no sting, just a meeting out of mutual friendship. Needless to say, the class and her teacher were astonished.

These experiences were many years ago and they have taught me to listen so much better to how Spirit speaks to us and to pay attention to what Spirit says. There are so many stories to share, but I will leave it at this for now. One view I hold is that each of us are a vessel through which Spirit can enter the world to teach and enlighten if we simply choose to say Yes.

I think from all that has been described above, some of you may have had your curiosity tweaked a bit to play in this world with your emerging clear vision and refined senses. Some of you have already been doing this for years, so you know the value. Keep spreading the word—you know, the pebble thrown into the pond with ripple effect.

Now begin to look at what's next for you. Some of you have perhaps discovered new ways to relate to your world, to design a life that is your choosing free of how others have decided how you should live it. It is indeed a rich tapestry we are weaving together. I can't wait for the rest of this book to manifest. You may recall that I am making this up as I go. I don't even know the title for Chapter 11 yet . . . but I will in a moment. You can do the same thing in your life—just make it up as you go and enjoy the ride. Have fun!

I remember once during my Airborne days with SF, I was about to jump out of the aircraft. As the Jumpmaster guided me into the door and took control of my static line, he looked at me and in all seriousness said, "And for God's sake, be careful!!" He was clearly having fun with me. I was having fun too. I love falling through the sky. I also went through HALO training—Military Free Fall. What an experience! The world looks so different from up there when you are about to join the sky, especially in the dark of night jumping out of a jet many thousands of feet up.

Chapter 11
YOU CAN GO ANYWHERE
WITH A MAP AND A COMPASS

I just made this title up, just now. It was probably my reference to my life in Special Forces and jumping out of planes in the last paragraph that helped crystallize it. It was a common expression in our unit, "Just give me a map and a compass and I can go anywhere." That's a true statement in the SF community, and I imagine within any Special Ops group. Now we have GPS and instant digital information available. I still appreciate knowing the old way just in case technology fails.

For many years I maintained that each of us have a built-in compass. I still do, and that all we needed to do was become sensitive to the electromagnetic lines of the earth and know exactly what direction we were facing without a compass. I was practicing this with my kids. I also brought it up in Mountain Medicine. I think this is possible with practice and refinement, a work in progress and still on my to do list.

For the sake of this chapter, where would you go if you could go anywhere, and how would you get there? We all have our inner maps of the terrain we desire to traverse in life, and our inner compasses. Are you willing to expand on this map and the means to get there? Let's develop this notion together and see what shows up.

Let us consider our journey this lifetime that we are taking together now— acknowledging this may be one of many lifetime journeys that some of us have taken together before—an interesting thought and not original with me either, as many have stated this. But for this lifetime now, I am curious where you would like to go, what do you want to see, what would you like to experience, what would you like your loved ones to experience? They too are on this journey with you. At least we can agree that your mother and father ushered you into this life and may be there now. There may be more, like the rest of your family, should you have one. There is also your expanded family, your community, the world. How do you wish to view all these humans in your life? What do you want to share with them?

Pretend you have a map of the world in front of you. Pretend also that you have a compass and know how to use it. You don't have to know the world as if you've been there already. Just imagine it and where you would like to go, what you would like to see, what you would like to do, how will you go about getting there?

If something showed up for you, what was it? If nothing showed up for you, why not? These are serious questions. If you recall, I am suggesting we all get proficient at making our life up. Practicing imagination and utilizing our intuition and other means of communication with Spirit, can be introduced to assist us.

To be perfectly clear, there is nothing wrong with choosing to go nowhere. Some people have never left the town they were born in or gone far from home ever. If that is your choice, that is perfect. If it is not your choice or desire but done out of fear yet with a sometimes longing for adventure or just stepping into another world briefly, I'm just suggesting you go for the gusto and risk it. Live your dream, or create one that appeals to you, and then live it. I have learned that too many of us feel boxed in by circumstances, by a cage with an open door but afraid to take flight.

I can hear a lot of justification as to why you are not flying free, living your dream, maybe even a fairly valid one. What I am suggesting is that you learn to free yourself from these shackles by first imagining it, just picture it. Visualize it. Then little by little perhaps something begins to show up. Remember to keep your eye on the prize.

This short chapter is intended only for you to consider your dreams and if not living them, to consider why not and what it would take to do so. Remember you can have dreams while awake or while asleep. There will be more said about dreams and dreaming later. This is just a primer, a starter, to become comfortable with the notion of dreaming your life into manifest reality.

Perhaps look into your built-in maps and inner compasses to find your way to your dreams. Oh, and start writing down your dreams as part of manifesting your map.

Chapter 12
TAKING THE ROAD LESS TRAVELED

This is a chapter of encouragement. It takes courage to choose a road less traveled. By choosing this book you have chosen a road less traveled. Why? Because choosing to make up your life as you desire it, as you dream it up out of nothing, takes courage, takes a willingness to be different, to not be part of the flock, like Jonathan Livingston Seagull (Richard Bach). *Jonathan chose to be different.*

Being part of the flock is not a bad thing, as it is a stepping-stone to not being part of the flock. As you step into the life you see for yourself, the one you are creating without the approval of others, is a big step. I believe it is a step we are all to take in our becoming, but at different stages, different appearances, different paces, different rhythms—all representing our unique expressions of Self.

Consider that in our daring to be different, to marching to the beat of our own drum, this grants courage to others to do the same in their own lives. This could lead to anarchy and complete disarray if living from an unconscious unenlightened place, from say, little ordinary self. A lot of humans do. But that's not our direction.

Here I am referring to this path less chosen as arising out of our Higher Self's vision. Do you see the difference? I believe there is an order and a cohesiveness to the Universe with a purpose even though it shows up as random. Recall the *Law of Entropy* wherein all things in the universe are seen as expanding and moving away from every other celestial entity, creating more distance from everything in this process of expansion.

I asked the Universe about this many years ago. I was concerned that perhaps we were headed to the experience of complete emptiness, no more stars to behold, dissolved into a vast expansiveness of infinity as everything moves away from everything else. Science has predicted this. Difficult to wrap our heads around.

The Universe answered me. It was not moving further and further apart from itself never to return. It was breathing. Breath in, breath out, for eternity. Expanding and contracting forever. Life emerging and dissolving over and over again, new forms, new everything, forever. Difficult to wrap my head around.

This however made more sense to me since that was how the Universe explained it to me. How do you see it?

Let's take a look at the road less traveled by each of us and what it means to us, and those in our sphere of life, our families, our communities, even the world, as this is part of our arena too—even when we do not feel we are impacting life on that large a scale. Consider that we are. Remember the pebble thrown into the pond of the universe notion and the ripples each of us create.

The road less traveled has been taken by many. And viewing their journeys and their teachings illuminates our lives and makes a difference, I believe. You will need to form your own opinion if you wish to weigh in on how you feel about this. If you intend to embark upon the road less traveled in your own life, perhaps it will become important to you that you consider this.

There is another expression for taking the road less traveled. I call it going upstream. I wrote on this notion a few years ago. I will include it below for your reading.

GOING UPSTREAM

There is a flow to the universe if someone looks at it. And there is an expression called *going with the flow*, implying an at-ease-ness when one chooses to go with the flow. And often one does not have this choice to go against the flow, or one does not make this choice. Or one consciously makes the choice to go against the flow . . . to go upstream. Why would anyone make that choice if it were easier to go downstream with the flow?

I don't know the answer to that other than to feel it is part of the human blueprint—that we are actually designed to go against the flow. The Buddha, Jesus, Mohammed, Krishna, and other Masters chose to go upstream. Lao Tzu, Gandhi, Yogananda, Amma, and many others chose to speak of that which was uncommon, to teach us—to go upstream. Einstein, Bohr, Tesla, Mother Teresa, Martin Luther King Jr, and too many more to name, spoke of living life in a better way and led us there through their words and their work. They too chose to go upstream. And it has made all the difference to the lives of so many that they did.

And from the point of view of water, it does not care where it is in the stream—whether it is upstream or downstream, or seeping into the earth of the streambed, or rising into the sky as it evaporates, it is still water. There is no direction to it, only beingness.

Life is a series of choices and expressions. Life can be participated in passively at times, and at times actively. But the truth is we human beings are always doing something even if it is nothing. We are always engaging with life or choosing not to—and regardless, we are still engaging with life even in our perceived non-engagement. Life can be viewed as a balancing thing, and we can be in balance with it or not. I now like to think of living life with effortless ease, in allowing whatever shows up in my particular path as a contribution to me, as an offering by Spirit which then challenges me and says, *"Now what do you want to do with this offering?"*

This may be what so many humans have been confronted with, who then accepted the challenge, coming to this decision . . . *"If I am human and aware that I am on this beautiful and amazing planet--our Mother Earth—with so many beings appearing in need of a better way, with so many appearing unable to see more clearly, while I perhaps have been blessed with better sight than some, then let me do something about it . . . I will go upstream. There are many places I can rest along the way, and I know I am in good company with the many who have gone before me, and the many who will perhaps notice and follow, and perhaps some who will join me. This is my choice . . . and Spirit is smiling."*

John Mills

In taking the road less traveled—or going upstream—I am suggesting that there is an element of risk involved. In embracing the unknown, in trying what has not been tried, in becoming comfortable with being uncomfortable, in being willing to step outside of yourself, you become a trail blazer, a pioneer of Spirit. You also become a light for others.

In being able to be with not knowing how something will turn out and doing it anyway takes a bigger you than you have been used to being. And we all have this capacity to show up in life this way. I am suggesting that we all take this on. The world is a troubled place. It needs more teachers of love, compassion, understanding, kindness, and whatever your Spirit calls you to be.

This has been a challenging chapter. It was a challenging chapter to write. Like the title, taking a road less traveled puts us exactly on that road. What does being on this road less traveled look like to you, to how you will live your life? This is worth careful thought and consideration. And consider the difference it will make to others.

Perhaps dare to be different . . . like *Jonathan Livingston Seagull*.

Chapter 13
POETIC REFLECTIONS

Everyone is a poet, you know. Perhaps some of us were once told by someone that we can't write; that we especially can't write poetry, that we can't do a lot of things, and unfortunately many of us believed that—we bought into someone else's assessment of what we can or cannot do.

I say we are all poets. That does not imply that we all desire to write poetry, but I clearly believe that we all can write poetry if we want to. If we think of poetry as saying something we wish to say about life, or about nature, about beauty, about feelings, about our Self, about anything, expressed in our own unique style, then we should do it. That is poetry.

It is like you do not have to be a Yogi to do Yoga. One definition of Yoga is that it is any activity done mindfully. That covers a much wider range. Recall that Yoga yokes the mind and the body. Everyone can do Yoga. Poetry may be any use of words done mindfully that expresses you, your feelings, your inner nature, your uniqueness, that you simply wish to put into words, as colorfully or artistically as you are called to do. It need not be for anyone but yourself. You may find however that your words will always touch someone beyond yourself. And they may touch many.

I never thought I was a poet until one day I decided I wanted to write a poem. I don't even remember what it was, but I did call it a poem. Then eventually one poem led to another and in time I considered myself a poet. And you may recall in an earlier chapter that I said I never wrote a poem but that poems were written *through* me— or maybe poems wrote me. It doesn't matter really as I still like writing them and sharing them from time to time.

I once hiked with a group of men who named themselves *The Undaunted Saunterers*. When I left the area to move from Oregon back to New Hampshire, it coincided with a backyard party that one of the guys arranged for all of us. I wrote a poem as a tribute to the men and read it to them and their guests at the party, capturing the essence of our hikes together. That poem, *To Be Undaunted*, appears below.

I like to capture special experiences in poetry too, like when I completed my Ayurveda training at Kripalu and a poem I wrote during the course, *When Old Souls Touch*, was selected for presentation at our graduation and I was asked to read it.

And then there was the time we completed the North Direction on the Medicine Wheel of the Shaman's Altar. Among our experiences we got to visit *the Lower World, the Middle World, and the Upper World*. It was an amazing journey we shared, and my partner, Carolina (Caro), originally from Ecuador, was the perfect partner. We discovered we shared previous lifetimes and were shamans in times past. This inspired me to write a poem about our experience which I later shared with our group traveling to Peru for training with the Q'ero in the Andes.

You will discover in the poem below *Journey to the North* that simply writing about that experience in prose wouldn't have captured the essence of the experience as colorfully as a poem would. You get to play more with poetry.

Recently I was asked by Susan, a High School classmate, to write a poem for our last class reunion. Hence, *Turning the Pages* was born and appears below.

And Nature and Love and magical things and good feelings especially inspire me too. Sometimes sadness or pain or hurt or loss need to be expressed and writing a poem about those qualities is for me a way of letting the experience go. And it often transforms the experience into something good, like part of the healing.

So, writing about these things poetically allows me more freedom to express feelings and more opportunity to play. I become my poems when I am writing them, and I get to be an Artist, and I always express gratitude for the unseen source behind them.

I will share a few with all of you here. Why? Because it is fun to share my poetry. It is like playing to me. And I get to share my art. And I get to be with each of you in a different way. So here goes . . .

TO BE UNDAUNTED

I am not delicate
Perhaps sensitive
A bit
But not delicates

Give me some mud on my boots
And some on my face too
A rain-soaked park
And too cold for comfort
Sometimes

I love Nature
I love grass and flowers and snow
I love trees . . .
And I love them fallen in my path at times
And to watch birds and deer and butterflies

I want skinned knees
Achy joints and sore back and muscles
From an arduous climb
I want to feel my walk

I want rough hands with callouses
From clearing trail
The sun on my face
And sunburn too

I want to get lost
And find my way
Most of the time
And enjoy being lost too

I want all the possibilities
All the experiences
That life offers
And then more

I want to get dirty
And sweaty
And struggle at times
I want torn pants or shirt or skin
From trying too hard
If it looks easy
I'll choose a different path
You'll often find me
On the road less travelled
You know . . .
The one most don't take

And I want my friends
On the trail with me
Often
And to be alone too

I want the wind in my face
And dust in my eyes
I want to fall sometimes
And get up again
With ease
Or not

I want to squint at the sunrise
And the sunset too
And bake in the noonday sun
And feel grateful

I want to behold a starry sky
And the darkness of a moonless cloud-shrouded night
Or a cool dense deep forest
And listen to the sounds of the soundless

As I get old
I want my wrinkles to have wrinkles
And I want them all smiling

I want to feel life
All of it—Everything!
And I want to wink at you
Why?

Because I am undaunted
And this is what I choose
This is what I do

. . .

WHEN OLD SOULS TOUCH

There are no words
to describe this . . .
this experience I hold

But inside the words
inside the feelings
there is something

Something that gathers
and contains
everything

It is pure and sweet
it is lovely and light
it is wildly delicious

It calls to me
and it begs
come into my heart

And so I do
smiling and entering
embracing spirit

All this I know
because I have touched
an old soul

JOURNEY TO THE NORTH

Like a hummingbird
you flew into my life
and landed
beside me

And our journey
(this time)
began again

We visited words
and worlds
unknown
to so many

Seeking our original faces
we found them
how colorful and beautiful you were
how happy and content was I
with so little . . . and the children

We rode the white Buffalo
walked through fire
were given our medicine names

We soared as eagles
glimpsed our becoming
and discovered love and joy
in our one heart

Playing in the ocean
we rode waves of eternity
and dissolved into them

We shed roles like robes
stories, fears, teachers too
we became invisible
and entered timelessness

We remembered we agreed to forget
and forgot to remember
so we could experience

In stillness we glided with Raven
on currents of wind
and tasted the sweet nectar
of life with Hummingbird

Stillness in motion
motion in stillness

We touched
each other's hearts
and slowed them
to the rhythm of Mother Earth

We sat at a table
prepared for us by our Shaman lineage
met our family
took our seats . . . and filled ourselves

Climbing a silver thread
we visited the Upper World
there Pachakuti allowed us a peek
at what lies ahead

As the veil parted
we saw the past, future
and now

Walking together in the circle of time
we saw us in the future
creating us now

We beheld creation
and each other
in a single breath of awareness

Now as we move towards our becoming
and the unknowable
we chose two words to bring home
with us Joy and Love

and became them
. . .

TURNING THE PAGES

For my class reunion

We are like the pages of a book
A good book
while it may appear we are nearing the end of a chapter
Perhaps even the end of the book to some
Consider we are not

Consider that we are just ready to begin
Writing a new one . . .
Chapter
Book
Whatever

What do you want to design
Compose
Be
Now

Just decide

Do you have a Play in mind
Do you have Play in mind
You see, this thing we call Future
Is up to each of us
To create and make up as we wish

If the one looking back at us from the mirror
Is not the one in our High School class photo
Consider it is
We have only grown in wisdom and life experience

And this has left a roadmap on our face

Each line is testament to our journey
Where has your journey brought you
And what would you share of it
With others
What gifts are yours to share
Do you wish to share any of it

There is no future
There is only NOW
Yesterday is a memory
Tomorrow lives only in imagination
It is only now that we are truly alive

What do we want to do with all these now moments
That lie before us
As we say goodbye to each other today
while greeting the next moment yet to be

This is worthy of thought

Is there a child
We wish to smile at or hug
Perhaps share a story with
What will you say
About the story of your life

Make it a good one
One that will make a difference
To that little life before you
As your story unfolds

Just like turning the pages of a good book

John Mills

Chapter 14
FROM HERE TO THERE AND BACK AGAIN

This title also appeared in *Lord of the Rings*. It's meaning may take on more in the context of this book and our lives, although there is clearly overlap. What we are all exploring together is getting there (somewhere) from here (where we are now). There may be no return for us—to the way we were—but we may find it necessary to recall our journey and who we were in order to show others the path we've taken. This is what pioneers and explorers do. They discover and then share what they've discovered. I see this as exciting. Maybe not all will, though I suspect that perhaps some of you will.

I see much of what is offered in the world today as going nowhere. I do understand there is purpose to every experience, but I also see that it is time to learn from our experiences. They have served to show us it is time to reconsider, regroup, and choose a better path. In other words, many of us have strayed from the trail, and some are headed over the cliff if we don't stop and change course. Does anyone see this occurring in life for anyone they know? If so, you know what I'm talking about. You may have even noticed this occurring for you, a direction you have taken that you now see as time to change. Do you recall an old proverb that says, *if we don't change the direction in which we are going, we will end up where we are headed? Where are you headed?*

And are you happy with where you are headed? If not, there is no better time than *NOW* to consider changing direction. You may notice this brings us full circle to the first chapter of this book, but we've all gotten to see a lot more since beginning. You can view this as *from here to there and back again.*

Chapter 15
AS WE HEAL WE REVEAL

Healing is an interesting word and worth understanding from many levels. I am a physician and studied health for most of my adult life and I am still not sure what healing is. I do understand a bit so I will share that with you.

In the usual sense of healing, like a wound, science still cannot explain it. We can observe what happens to damaged tissue and all the stages of healing, from gross observation to microscopic and subcellular. We do not understand why healing happens. It appears the body has an innate propensity to recreate itself in its original form whenever it deviates from that original blueprint. But why does that happen? What makes this occur? Let's explore this.

We know that a holographic image of any part of a tree contains an image of the whole tree. Perhaps the tree reproduces itself along the image of this blueprint. It doesn't matter if leaves are blown off or branches break. New ones replace them.

We also know certain species regrow parts—like salamanders grow new tails, lobsters regrow claws, to name a few—yet we humans have not learned this. If we lose part or all of an extremity, hand, arm, leg, it's gone. Yet the imprint remains. We call this imprint the phantom limb experience. We can even measure its energetic presence. Yet we have not learned the ability to re-inhabit that energic phantom limb appendage with flesh and blood. Why not?

When I was very young, I actually considered this and wondered why not? I knew then that salamanders and lobsters could do this. I used to think that if we could imagine this hard enough, we could do it. I still believe this. But for the moment, let's stick to the healing we can observe and then work from there.

So what we think we understand is our observation of the healing process. If we get cut—sustain a laceration—this can be sutured when big enough, or just left to heal on its own when superficial. Even deep wounds heal on their own although may not appear like our skin or muscle used to appear. The point being made here is healing occurs with or without our help. There are exceptions.

Exceptions include but are not limited to when we lose a part of our self—like an amputation—or have a very complicated messy or dirty wound that can get in the way of optimal healing or even cause our health to deteriorate by way of infection or incapacity, even death. This may become a difficult chapter, but I will do my best to stick to simplicity. I will be discussing some perhaps uncommon notions here yet intend to communicate them in as simple and understandable manner as I can, simply because I prefer simple over complex or complicated or obtuse.

Healing is an extremely important aspect of life. To heal well and easily greatly contributes to the quality of our life. I hope we can all agree on that. Note that the first four letters of healing and the first four letters of health, is *heal*. At the risk of sounding simplistic, I do want to draw your attention to key points. This is one.

This chapter will evolve in an order that will eventually give you an idea of how comprehensive and important this concept of healing is in our lives on the usual levels we commonly think of—physical, mental, emotional—but also includes healing at a soul level, as well as the energetic and spiritual planes of life. They are all related. We'll build this slowly. For the purpose of understanding something extremely important in life, slow and simple are two of my touchstones.

I will discuss things that I feel facilitate healing as well as the things that hinder it. While I have a background in healthcare, I want to mention that probably most of us can come up with nearly the same list I do. You see we all have a good idea of this stuff already. It will get a little dicier as we move into the mental and emotional realms, and even more so when entering the energetic realm. But really, it's not that complicated, and my intention is to make this easy and understandable. Even when we move into discussion on quantum theory, I want to keep it simple and flowing without a lot of eyerolling and head scratching. You'll see what I mean when we get there. Isn't this fun, really?!

I especially enjoy that we are on this journey together on Spaceship Earth. It is not only possible, but entirely probable, that some great things will come out of this voyage together. Perhaps a sequel to this book should be us contributing our stories of what showed up in our lives after engaging with life at this level. There is great power in community and sharing powerful experiences. Somehow most newspapers and tabloids seldom capture that on their pages. Let us do it then.

Important to good healing is good health. Seems obvious but often not considered. Healthy tissues heal better. Many of us do not inhabit bodies that are healthy. Have you seen any? If so, you know what I'm talking about. Are you one perhaps?

I can speak to this as both a physician and someone who has inhabited an unhealthy body in the past. Chronic stress, toxic work environment (not patients but colleagues), poor diet, inconsistent sleeping patterns and often not enough sleep— the usual contributions that many of us experience in being less than well.

Does anyone identify with this pattern? If not, do you have your own impediments to good health? If you have none, you can help me write this book. I won't say skip the book because I think we could have a rich discussion that could benefit many, much like my intention in writing this book in the first place.

The first thing to acknowledge is to examine what we think constitutes good health. As I mentioned in the introduction to this book, it depends on the individual. However, to serve as a benchmark for comparison on where each of us weigh in on this question I will submit the following Ayurvedic definition of good health that I alluded to in the Introduction as well.

Sama dosah samagris ca sama dhatu mala kriyah prasannamendriya manah vastha ityabhidhiyate (Sanskrit from Sushruta Samhita 15.38). It means, *One who is established in self (knows oneself thoroughly), who has balanced doshas (our constitution qualities), balanced agni (whole body digestive fires), properly formed dhatus (tissues), proper elimination of malas (waste products), well-functioning bodily processes, and whose mind, soul and senses are happy is called a healthy person.*

We can see that this interpretation of health is a departure from how most of us think of good health in the West as *merely the absence of disease.* Think of this Sanskrit Ayurvedic version as more comprehensive. So, are you still healthy?

If you can look into your Self, see what is there for you. What is healthy? What appears unhealthy? Use your intuition or your ability to communicate with all of your body parts and with your mental/emotional bodies, and with your soul too.

What shows up for you? Be honest and genuine. This is only for you. No one is grading you. No consensual reality—the reality of others—gets a vote.

And if you don't really know what is healthy and what is unhealthy, keep looking, keep practicing. It will surface. There will be clues. There are always clues if you are looking.

As the heading of this chapter suggests, **As We Heal We Reveal**, and this is on many levels, and from different perspectives, the obvious and the not-so-obvious. We reveal more of what we are looking at and for. We also begin revealing more of who we are to the world—to how we show up in life.

As toxic residue melts away and leaves our body, as we detoxify our physical, mental, and emotional bodies, as our souls heal, we see so much clearer the healing path ahead for us and we appear different to the world that surrounds us. We also draw different experiences and different people into our spheres of existence. We attract different energies. I will let these thoughts settle in with you for a minute. Think about them. You do not need to buy into them, just consider them before moving on to the next paragraph.

To give you a hint at how subtle this process can be, consider an Ayurvedic piece of wisdom that says, if we eat in a state of anger, or with someone who is expressing anger, blame, hostility, we take that emotional energy into our body and into our mental and emotional bodies as well. This then builds up toxicity in those areas, poisoning us.

This is true of the food we eat too from an Ayurvedic point of view, really from any energetic point of view from any ancient wisdom source. If an animal is treated badly or killed inhumanely before it appears on our table to eat, that energy is transferred to us. This may not make sense to you. I'm just suggesting you can consider that it is more than a physical world of nuts and bolts in which we live. It is also one of feelings, emotions, thoughts, vibrational energies of many kinds, all interacting with our own systems in a beneficial or potentially toxic way.

I wish I could claim this is an original idea of mine—my ego would love that—but my Self wouldn't if it wishes to be in integrity. These notions have been around forever, and written about, and spoken about long before the written word. Add this to your bag of things to consider as we tell the rest of the story. And of course . . . don't believe a word I say. Accept this idea or reject it as you see fit. If accepted, practice it and see what shows up for you. See what shifts for you.

Are you beginning to see a pattern here, the circular pattern of returning to our Selves, the relatedness and connections between everything we uncover together? I have stated before, and will again, everything is related to everything else. Just for the fun of it, make a short list of everything we have discussed so far and see how many ideas, concepts, qualities, you can connect with all the other ideas, concepts, qualities. There is overlap always if you look with an inquiring mind. And I know all of you have inquiring minds and are learning to operate consistently in life from a state of mindfulness, or already do.

This is a key point by the way. Live in a state of mindfulness as much as possible. Be aware of the moment. Be aware of *Now*. It is the only moment we are alive. We have the memory of being alive yesterday. We have the hope of being alive tomorrow. But it is only in this very moment now that we are alive. Learn from Sewar Kenti (Hummingbird) and Ohmaak Aistoo (Raven) about *timelessness*, about *stillness in motion, motion in stillness*. And then take flight in this realm yourself.

Later in this book we will talk about stretching out this moment of experience we call *Now* into eternity. This is what Raven and Hummingbird teach us. They teach us about the experience of timelessness. Sounds intriguing, doesn't it?

If you are looking for more of an explanation as to *When We Heal We Reveal*, consider that you already have it. Spend a moment with your Self and see what presents itself. You should be getting pretty good at this by now. Perhaps right now just write down 10-20 ways to heal, and another 10-20 things that you feel are in the way of healing. Look over the items you came up with. You can name a bunch more if you wish. Then be with each list. Which do you choose for yourself and for your loved ones? So now, what's stopping you from including all the healthy ones your Self came up with. What's stopping you from dropping the unhealthy ones. You see, you don't even need me.

If anyone came up with only ways to heal and you are practicing all of them and have no things in the way of healing—i.e. nothing is blocking your path to complete and vibrant health, you too can help me write this book.

Let's break it down some more. There are things that we can identify that nourish our physical bodies. You probably have a bunch on the list you just created on the ways of healing. Likewise, there are things we can identify that nourish our mental and emotional bodies that address our psychological wellbeing—equally as important as our physical wellbeing, yet with differences and with overlap. We will look at soul healing and energetic healing and the role Spirit plays after that.

How do we nourish our physical bodies? One of the first things that comes to mind for me is the food we eat. I should mention that I love food, love to eat good food, and have brought little discrimination to the choice of foods I've eaten over the years when young. I got away with this pattern for a long time because I have always been healthy and fit and active and recognized no limitations. But unhealthy patterns leave clues—just like success does.

Our bodies and our cells and all the machinery that runs a human being are miracle workers, when we truly look at the incredible number of functions performed every nanosecond in a single cell, not to mention in the system as a whole. Yet even our bodies and all its parts need care and maintenance, just like our mental and emotional states and our souls. This care begins first with an awareness that we in fact need to maintain our systems well for optimal health.

We need to become not only vigilant at what keeps our machinery running smoothly but become sensitive to all the fine nuances and sensations and feelings when it begins to run less smoothly. There are clues everywhere, easily noted when we pay attention, when we listen in, to what our bodies are telling us. Our bodies truly know what they need and are constantly trying to get our attention. Most of the time most of us are too busy to listen. I was one of those people.

Not paying attention over a long time ultimately becomes a pathway to disease, debility, (self) destruction, and death. This can all be prevented if we effectively intervene in a timely manner. There are many ways we can intervene effectively.

And our bodies can be so forgiving. They can be pretty far down the road to ill health and still recover fully when we take an interest and start caring for them.

Starting with food, and specifically with our choices of the food we eat, let's deepen this inquiry. Remember this is all from my point of view, and you know what you can do with my point of view . . . don't trust it. But perhaps do consider it at least.

It is important to know that there are literally hundreds of thousands of papers written on just nutrition alone every year. Some of them offer very different points of view and perspectives. Many contradict one another. It can be mind-boggling! How do you know what to trust or believe or follow?

The simple answer is don't trust any of it. It makes you crazy when you look at all the opinions on how YOU should do it. This is nothing more than consensual reality trying to sound its intelligent best to buy you out, to take over your thinking, to sell you something. I will offer you some simple guidance here which may help.

And this is not to suggest that you should not study something of value. Education and gaining knowledge can be very important. When the material starts making you crazy, that's a sign. Back off. Just be wary of buying into anything if it goes against your better judgment or intuitive self, against your gut feeling. You will know the difference eventually but get good at practicing this and trusting your internal guide.

We all have a built in BS meter. Do I need to interpret BS for you? And remember, we are all unique. I strongly encourage all of us to trust our Selves in this matter. Remember Tony Robbins' suggestion to just look at your food and ask, "Is this going to cleanse me or clog me?" That's a hint. We know. And when we don't know, we can ask our Selves for the answer.

In the area of *Food*, I first want to point out that much of what we eat, is in fact not food. It is packaged and sold in stores, so we think it is food. But when we read the label and ingredients, we are immediately informed that it is a compilation of many chemicals and things made to look like food and taste like food but is really not food or fit to eat. Or if it once was food in its original natural state when picked, most of the life and nutrition has been removed from it during its processing before going into a box or a can. This is the stuff we then put in our bodies that adds more to its toxicity than to its maintenance of healthy bodily functions or recovery when healing is called for. *Rule#1 is Be careful what you call food.* So much of it isn't.

My guidance—which I follow for myself—in the area of food is to eat natural, eat organic when possible (despite all the press about this—my take on this is that pesticides just aren't good for humans). Eat a clean diet. Eat fresh fruits and vegetables, seasonal when

112

possible as Ayurveda and other wisdom sciences teach. Avoid junk food. We all know what junk food is. If not, look it up and see how it is defined and depicted.

You may recall a book a while ago that suggested shopping just the perimeter of your grocery store. That's where all the fresh produce hangs out—fruits, vegetables, eggs, dairy, meat, etc. It also suggested that all the stuff in the center aisles were processed and packaged in boxes or cans, nutritionally depleted, and to skip most of it. Also, if you can't pronounce the ingredients, or if the list is too long to bother reading, don't bother reading it, and don't buy it. Simple guidelines. This accommodates my preference for simplicity. I also believe this happens to be better for our bodies and our health.

Non-food can cause inflammation in the body. More specifically stated, the process of digestion of non-food creates free radicals in our system. That is, a lot of what we eat causes an inflammatory reaction in our gut resulting in so-called leaky-gut syndrome. Our inner lining of our intestines is only one cell thick. Inflammation produces damage to this lining—think of it as tiny holes appearing from this damage that then allow the bad stuff (free radicles among other things) of what we eat to pass into our blood stream and get transported throughout our bodies.

These are toxins and by-products of digestion of non-foods that then serve as a source of inflammation, ultimately damaging our healthy cells and tissues if not altered by introducing a healthy diet. This is not Bio-Physiology 101. This is just smart and should become common sense for us. However, please note that *common sense* is not so common these days. Make it a point to educate yourself in this area. Real food is important to really good health. It is wise to make this our second nature. Our gut-brain thinks so too.

It is interesting what Ayurveda has to say about food, the qualities of the variety of foods we eat, and the effect of food on our body. There is even seasonal advice. This is worth looking into. It is also interesting to note that Ayurveda identifies processed white sugar and processed white flour as toxins. In other words, go natural or

113

wholegrain when using any sweetener or grain products. In a restaurant, ask for this, or bring your own if you feel so motivated.

In a nutrition course for health professionals that I took at Kripalu taught by a PhD Nutritionist that studied this a lot, he suggested that all humans have a gluten sensitivity—some of this clinically significant (like in coeliac disease), some not so. He suggested that during the week we were together to eat only a gluten-free diet from Kripalu's dining room, which offered a wide variety of healthy foods. His point was that the introduction of grains into the human diet was relatively recent on an evolutionary time scale and many of us still had sensitivities to them. Most of us volunteered to try it. I was not aware of a gluten sensitivity for myself. Still I felt better that week as did all the rest volunteering to try gluten-free eating. Maybe another clue?

If you eat meat, eating grass-fed beef is better than not. Cost may be a factor. Just decide how much you value your health. You can always cut back on quantity or eat different proteins that also support creating a healthy body. Avoid cutting back on quality. You can but it may show up in your body. Just consider how much you are worth. Are you really invested in taking care of the temple in which you dwell?

You may have heard that many (if not all) of our streams, rivers, lakes and oceans are polluted, or fast becoming seriously polluted, so much so that even fish can't live in some of them anymore. Consider this when consuming fish, usually a healthy source of protein, and fish oils are beneficial to our brain tissue. The size of the fish matters if from the sea. Large fish are known to have higher quantities of mercury in them. As always, educate yourself about your options.

You may also consider while becoming more conscious of the foods we eat, of working the other side of the aisle too. Become an advocate for cleaning up our environment and minimizing pollution on a global scale. Begin slowly but realize that this is vitally important to our health and to the health of our planet in the long run—quickly becoming thought of as the *short run* given the timeframe we have to accomplish this. At least think about it and consider beginning somewhere in tiny bits—the pebble thrown into the pond theory creating ripples that spread outward. One person can make a difference. Why wait?!

On the subject of water, drink lots of it too, to keep the system flushing out toxins— filtered is very good, through a charcoal filter, and reverse osmosis if available. Distilling your own water is another good option. Avoid tap water that is treated with chemicals. I believe chlorination and fluorination are not good for us. Others will differ with this opinion. It's okay. You choose.

By the way, I am constantly reminding myself to drink more water even when I know the value of doing so.

And a few more words on food, specifically *fun food*, also known as comfort foods. These are not always our healthiest choices from a physical nutritional point of view but consider that they perhaps nourish our mental and emotional states, not to mention the soul. To this Ayurveda says, all things in moderation. Afterall, let's remember that we are human, and it is up to each of us how we do this journey to a glowing healthy vital life. No one size fits all. Introducing rigidity into our thinking and our behavior may not be wise. You decide for yourself.

Clues will show up as to whether we are being successful at this or not. Then it is up to each of us to recognize it and alter course as we see best. Remember, the key is increasing awareness and mindfulness in all things.

Let's look at nutrition for our mental and emotional states next. I realize all these areas could be given separate chapters, but I want to emphasize that health and healing and how we nourish ourselves are intimately related. We will return to more discussion on them as individual topics later.

How many of you are aware that we have already covered ways to nourish our mental and emotional bodies? That's right. We more than touched upon them earlier, in the importance of reducing stress and tension in our lives via calming our systems down with meditation, Yoga, mindful exercise, joy-producing experiences, etc. Do you recall this now?

How we eat and what we eat and when we eat plays a role too. In Ayurveda, there are rajasic foods that wire us, make us hyperactive, more restless. There are tamasic foods that slow us down, create lethargy, or put us asleep after eating. Then there are sattvic foods that produce harmony and calm in the body. Explore these in your Ayurvedic research. It is quite well explained and simple to follow.

This is true for where we choose to live as well. Fast paced busy city life (or work environment, or anything else very busy or fast-paced) leads to a *rajasic* tension- filled or stressful experience that our bodies and mental states then absorb. Living in a *sattvic*, or harmonious environment, is nourishing for our minds and bodies. Climate plays a role too. All this is related.

Now for the fun of it, come up with your own ideas of what would introduce more harmony in your life, more calm, less stressful experiences. This can be dietary, home and family life, work environment, where you live, how you think and react in general. Be creative in coming up with ideas. Just remember you are going for experiences and expressions of harmony.

Consider an example of seeing an argument taking root. You may choose to stick in there as it escalates and gets worse. No winners. You feel worse afterward. Or if you saw it coming, perhaps you didn't need to be right about it to soothe your ego, and just stopped it, walked away agreeing to talk later when you both cooled off a bit, whatever. I've been there, the one who didn't walk away, and it got worse to my (our) detriment. It just wasn't worth it. Just an example. You can come up with your own. You can come up with many, I'm sure. But you get the idea.

It's like eating when you are angry as mentioned earlier. You take this energy into your body from the experience. Food is one vehicle to nourish us or perhaps injure us, energetically or chemically. Do you see how many levels there are of this to consider? You don't need to bother, but it may guide you to a better experience of yourself. You get to choose again.

I often mention to my patients in the appropriate context that there are two types of stress (to keep it simple). I grab myself by my collar and begin to pull on it firmly, stating, *"This is when stress has you, dragging you all around the room."* Then I release that hold, point to where it was, move my finger to under my arm as if I'm embracing my stress, and then state, *"Or you can befriend it, as if it has something to say to you, perhaps teach you something. The same stress, it didn't go away, you only changed your relationship with it. Now it is your friend."* Most of my patients get it . . . maybe all of them do. They seem to understand they do not need to be at the ill effect of the thing they call stressful.

Practice this, nourishing your mental and emotional bodies. You can read more about it too but try to stick to your own discovery of it. There may be wisdom here for you to discover. This area can appear vast, or you can simplify it so it works for you and adds to your life in a highly beneficial way.

Let's move onto nourishing one's soul now. This is where the *dicier* comes in mentioned above. Perhaps not all of us even acknowledge the existence of a soul although almost all of us have heard it mentioned before. Is that accurate?

So, I will share my experience with you all in the light of this being just a good (hopefully) novel and I'm being a storyteller. And if it makes sense, try it on. Just words and ideas, remember? It's up to you how you play with them and bring life to them for your Self.

I have encountered the mention of the Soul in many theatres—It was in my Yoga training, my Ayurvedic training, my Shamanic training, not to mention it commonly mentioned in numerous books I've read, meetings and courses I've attended, and in my early experience attending Sunday school and church as a young person. Perhaps the word Soul is common to most of us. I will leave it up to each of us to define it for ourselves, or not, if there is nothing there for you. I will offer a brief description of my experience of Soul and you can consider the rest for yourself.

I will keep it simple. I think of soul as that part of our being that is eternal, the part of us that does not die when we surrender our physical bodies each lifetime. It is what we take with ourselves for eternity, or until we make the conscious choice to merge with the *One,* with all of Cosmic energy, surrendering our individuality to become *One with Spirit*. This was introduced to me by one of my instructors in my Ayurvedic training, an Ayurvedic physician and Guru from India. He told us that it did not matter whether we believed it or not, that it was so anyway :)

According to Shamanic wisdom, during the performance of the death rites, a Shaman trained in this experience, has the ability to not only see the soul leaving the body at the time of death but assists its departure and facilitates its journey into the unseen world of Spirit. With careful measurements, the soul has weight— a body with the soul present weighs slightly more than when the soul has just left. Don't take my word for this. Read about it, study it if interested, experience it the best you can, and form your own opinion.

Not only does the soul carry with it the memories of past lifetimes and all past experiences, it carries with it karmic and ancestral imprints from prior lifetimes. These often show up in our current lifetime in a variety of experiences. One such carried-over experience is when there is a family history of, for example, cancer or heart disease over generations, and then it shows up in your present family. Modern science has its own explanation for this hereditary pattern. Ancient Shamanic wisdom has another. You can pick one or make up your own.

On the subject of soul retrieval, again from a Shamanic perspective, one can leave parts of one's soul somewhere else due to traumatic life experiences. I have a friend who was born in Barcelona, then moved to Paris shortly after her fiancée and her father died in the same year. She studied Yoga in Paris for 4 years, later married an American and moved to the United States. Due to mounting difficulties with her experience of living in America and far from her homeland, she explored soul retrieval with a Shaman.

Eventually my friend determined that her move here was so traumatic that she left part of her soul behind. In doing this work, she recovered it and it changed her experience of life with this soul work and added understanding. Consider this an interesting story but with no scientific basis and no real merit and no way to confirm . . . or the

118

real thing. In any case she felt it benefited her life, so does it really matter to anyone else?

A Shaman identifies these past traumatic imprints carried over from lifetimes past, or from a current lifetime experience, as an energetic *splinter*. The Shaman's work is to locate it, and then remove that splinter, freeing that person of the need to carry this traumatic event with them any longer. This is said to produce a healing effect, and also frees up future generations from having to bear that imprint any longer. You can study this if interested.

I only mention a Shamanic approach to healing to point out the variety of ways we interpret dis-ease in our bodies and ways we can heal it. There are many. The field of energy medicine is rich with stories and experiences—and successful results. If you are open to it, there may be something there for you.

You will notice that I occasionally mention previous lifetimes. Not all of us are comfortable with this notion. That's okay. That's when you can just read this as a good story and be entertained or enlightened as you see fit and find value in some of the health tips offered otherwise.

The notion of reincarnation—that our souls re-inhabit a new and different body lifetime after lifetime for the purpose of soul growth through a variety of life experiences on our way to enlightenment and liberation—has been around since the first ancients and seers spoke of it. To any of you whose religion or personal philosophy does not align with this belief, and which you cannot support, it is okay. Just acknowledge your choice of free will and carry on. To me there is irrefutable evidence that we live many lifetimes on this journey of the soul.

Speaking of one of my own experiences during a past-lives reading with Caroline Myss, a well-known writer and speaker on an international level, she knew nothing about me when I first met her. I lived in Keene, NH at the time, and she lived in Walpole, NH about 16 miles north of Keene.

Caroline has done much work on intuitive diagnosis and healing and in those years was working closely with Neurosurgeon Norm

Shealy, the founder of the American Holistic Medical Association. As a footnote here, Caroline had three clients who survived AIDS back when everyone was dying from this condition. She referred to her three survivors as *White Crows*. Reading any of her books could be quite informative. At least they were for me. I consulted her for a past-lives reading because I was curious, having never had one before, and I heard she was good.

As she began that evening in her home where I visited her, she started out by saying, "Oh, this is interesting. I see you have had many lifetimes as a healer, and many lifetimes as a warrior. And this lifetime you combined the two." As I mentioned she knew nothing about me as we began.

Caroline did not know that I was a physician working in the Emergency Department at the then Cheshire Hospital in Keene, and that I was also in the US Army with Special Forces, commonly referred to as the Green Berets then. She also shared that I was active at the time of Jesus and Francis of Assisi, and that I had a number of lifetimes as a *Snow Indian* (her exact words)—Lakota, and other northern plains tribes. She did not know at the time that I strongly resonated with Native American culture and with Nature and the land the Native Americans lived off of and with, in harmony. She did not know that I shared a similar respect for and relationship with the land and with everything that lived upon it then. But what she said made perfect sense to me. It was a *knowing* for me.

Just listen to this as an interesting story, much like story tellers the world over tell at times. And if it opens a window of interest into other worlds for you, that's wonderful. And if not, that's fine too. I have nothing to sell you or convince you of other than offering you a deeper exploration of your Self in its many dimensions and levels.

This brings us to a discussion of Spirit. I leave it up to each of us to determine what Spirit means to each of us, or perhaps nothing at all for some of you. Again I have nothing to convince you of and I am not attached to any one perception or interpretation of what Spirit means to any one of us. I do have my own understanding and relationship with Spirit, and it is from this understanding that I offer what I am about to share.

For me, there is nothing we have to do to heal or nourish Spirit, so this conversation departs from ways we choose to nourish our physical, emotional, mental bodies and our souls that dwell within. Rather it is Spirit that nourishes and nurtures us and our experience of each of these domains in our lives. The more we are open to Spirit, the more we are consciously nourished and nurtured by Spirit. Clues are everywhere when we are looking.

As was mentioned earlier on these pages, you can interchange the word Spirit with Source, God, All There Is, Cosmic or Universal Intelligence, whatever feels comfortable for you. The label is not important, the experience is. *Knowing* is more important than *knowledge* of information. How you arrive at *knowing* from *knowledge of facts* is up to you. If you believe in nothing else beyond yourself— that is, no Spirit or God in your life—it is okay too. I wish you well on that journey too. There is no wrong path.

I experience Spirit as everywhere and in everything, connecting all things to each other simultaneously. It is intelligent. It is love. It is us and all of life in all its expressions. I will leave it up to each of you to discover what Spirit means in your life and how you wish to be with Spirit. Again, there is no wrong way.

For some closing comments on nourishing our Selves, physically, mentally, emotionally, and our Souls, I would like to stir the pot even more. Remember, this is the Advanced Course in which you are engaged. I will at times present something that may appear to be a contradiction to something stated previously. This will be one of them.

I believe there are many levels of awareness, levels of consciousness, other realities, even so-called parallel universes, that exist simultaneously with the one we are currently experiencing. I don't know. Just suppose this is true for now just for the fun of it :)

It has also been observed by physicists and others who study energy and our vibrational states, that when we vibrate at a certain frequency, we draw other experiences to us that are of similar vibrations, and we do not particularly draw things to us of substantially higher or lower vibrational frequencies. Perhaps we even repel such things that don't share our vibrational energies—like the opposing ends of two magnets when brought in proximity to each other, they repel each other. I don't know. But I do encourage us all to think about this to facilitate explaining the sometimes unexplainable.

The earth is an electromagnetic field. Even in high school I used to consider, what if we simply had an antigravitational field aboard our space craft—such that we could oppose the gravitational pull of the earth and just be repelled off the surface into space very rapidly. No fuel, just opposing magnetic forces, doing as we can demonstrate what opposing magnetic forces do. This may be simplistic and absurd to you scientists reading this, but crazier ideas have taken hold. Just something to consider.

What does this have to do with nourishing our bodies and minds? Perhaps if we utilize our energies well, think a certain way, manifest in a certain way, we can simply be immune and impervious to any offending or toxic substance that enters our energy field by eating it, drinking it, breathing it, swimming in it, and therefore nothing toxic will have any adverse effect on us. Practice this if you feel like it. I have been for some time and the experiences are interesting, the results affirming. Let me know what shows up for you. I'll include it in my next book. This is how we can work together and then share the bounty with others.

This brings this chapter *As We Heal We Reveal* to an end. I believe the challenge before us is to become more aware, more conscious of, the relatedness of all things mentioned above, and much perhaps that hasn't been mentioned. The unsaid things will be part of your personal exploration and discovery. There is no end to this journey we are on. If I can open a few doors for us to walk through, a few windows for us to peek through, this perhaps offers each of us a glimpse of the grand experience of life beyond that which we currently perceive.

Chapter 16
AND NOW WHERE FROM HERE

Before we begin the next chapter, I would like each of you to imagine how you would continue from here. What would you like to say as you write the rest of this story from here on? By now you are all getting pretty comfortable with what we are creating together here, maybe even recognizing the playful and imaginative quality to it. You have also heard me tell you that I'm making this all up from my introduction to this book.

Now I would encourage you all to start making it up too—start making up how you would like to be healthier, more vital, more mindful, more filled with joy, and how would you go about creating for yourselves and your loved ones more loving kindness, compassion and understanding, *and fun*—and then paying it forward.

In addition to making it all up, as in *pure fiction*, start thinking about the artist you wish to be for the rest of your life. It is entirely okay to change your path—your work, your career, your field of interest or endeavor, your form of artistic expression—at any time, to totally re-invent your Self into something entirely new and different that totally excites you and inspires you. You don't have to either. Just know that you can, even if it appears challenging, even if it looks impossible. Just ask anyone who has accomplished the impossible. Many have. Many have transcended *"it can't be done"* and did it.

I will request that each of you really be with this for a few moments or longer before moving onto the next chapter. We will continue the rest of our journey from there.

Chapter 17
THE RAINBOWS WE ARE

I just want to remind all of us that we are as colorful as a rainbow and to consider what a rainbow is in our world of what we see. First you need rain (water), and some clouds, and some sunshine, to create the image of a rainbow, and that it represents a reflection of the sunlight passing through the water droplets in the air creating a prismatic effect for our visual sensory organs—our eyes. Does anyone know why they show up as curved or arched?

Consider that rain is water of course, and that clouds are states of evaporated water—the darker the cloud the greater the water content. Sunshine is light from the sun. The rainbow is a combination of this light and water in the air. Simple ingredients for such beauty.

Perhaps a rainbow is not so brilliant or colorful on the energetic plane—a bunch of vibrations at a particular band of wave lengths that makes color visible to us. Perhaps it is even more brilliant or colorful on the energetic level. I don't know. But it is a good time to appreciate what we as so-called mere mortals are gifted by virtue of our humanness and our sensory organs.

We are of course far more than mere mortals, but we humans are often called this. I believe we in fact are immortal, or more accurately, our souls are. We go on and on and on as I mentioned in Chapter 15, retaining all our memories and experiences forever, unconsciously for most of us—yet they are recorded and there. As we clear out the mist, see beyond the veil, we begin to observe that which we forgot. I am not alone on this notion either. Far smarter and wiser humans than me agree on this. You'll have to discover the validity for yourself, or simply disregard it. Only words and ideas, remember?

The lesson in the rainbow, in all its beauty and simplicity, is that we humans are also pretty simple in terms of our components yet look at the amazing way in which we show up as living breathing organisms with hearts and minds and souls. Where does all this other stuff come from added to the basic components?

If we accept that we live in a sea of energy, that everything is energy, that we are energy, and that there is an intelligent organizing principle behind it, then it is simple. Getting to accept this and see this may be a stretch for some. I am just suggesting we each consider it.

So, there are those of us who may fully embrace this notion of our world of energy and of our very existence as pure intelligent energy and pure consciousness. For those of us who find it difficult at this time to see yourself as a being of intelligent energy, I only request that you stay open to the possibility that our physical and objective reality is only a tiny part of the experience of life.

You see, rainbows are not actually real things. They are illusions combining the right set of ingredients mentioned above. It is the same for us humans. We are not actually real things, as we too are illusions manifested out of our unseen world of energy. On an energy map we may show up as a variety of waveforms, varying shapes, sizes, configurations, vibrational frequencies, and not appearing human at all. Your class photo reports different images. The field of Quantum Mechanics explains this very well.

There is a story when a while back Albert Einstein and Niels Bohr, both renowned physicists, noted for their extraordinary work in quantum theory, were walking at night. A conversation about the moon ensued. Einstein maintained the moon was there whether we viewed it or not. Niels Bohr said it wasn't. It only appeared to be there because of the vibrations it emitted for our receptive sense organs to perceive it as such. Without going into detail, it was subsequently determined that Niels Bohr won that argument. Things are not really there just because they appear to be.

Include in this view the fact that astronauts walked on the surface of the moon. It is real in our physical and manifested world of experience, but in the world of energy there is far more empty space between the atoms of things appearing solid, than the material stuff (atoms and subatomic particles) comprising solid appearing things. I only want to touch on this subject to share some other ideas on our existence and our reality as we perceive it. This just reveals a glimpse of the great mystery and the many levels of realities that we may encounter in life.

This is a perfect segue into the next discussion of our *Rainbowness*. I recently watched a movie called The Time of the Sixth Sun. It was about global awakening and I highly recommend it. During the movie—which represented people all over the world and acknowledged the contribution of indigenous populations the world over—it was stated that it takes all of us to come together for the future of our planet, the red, the yellow, the black, and the white people from all over the world.

These individuals that are accepting this responsibility, awakening to it, and carrying the message of uniting all of us with each other for the common good of Mother Earth and all her beings are called **Warriors of the Rainbow.** I like that. I think nothing more need be said about it for now. Are you a Warrior of the Rainbow? If you don't see yourself as that, are you willing to become one?

What this quality simply represents, and states, is that we are doing almost irreparable harm to our planet and our only home if we don't change direction. It will take a strong, united, conscious effort for all of us to come together to save the planet as we know it.

There may be much resistance from those in power and with great wealth who want to preserve the status quo of their existence, or even increase their power and wealth to the detriment of many others and to our earth. Fortunately, even people of power and wealth are waking up to what is needed and stepping out to reverse what mankind has wrought over many years. This will take time and many rainbow warriors. The time to begin is now. What would you like to do for your part?

This will also take a balancing of feminine and masculine energies and principles, perhaps a merging of both as we each possess these qualities within ourselves. Coming into balance for all of us may be one of the greatest challenges for restoration of health—for humans, for our planet, for anything. All of the great wisdom sciences of the world speak of the importance of balance. Where are we out of balance? Have we even looked? Are we willing to, and then are we willing to do something to restore balance and health? And if we find this is of value and works for us, are we then willing to pay it forward? We are all in this together. It will perhaps benefit everyone when we engage ourselves in this work.

PART II
Qualities of Being Essential to Achieving Great Health

QUALITIES OF BEING

Introduction to Part II

What follows next is a deeper look into the qualities of living that are known to many but practiced in depth by few. Keep in mind that on a planet with nearly eight billion people, a *few* is still a lot of people. This will be an opportunity for each of us to examine these qualities and decide whether we are practicing them and weaving them into every aspect of our waking or sleeping life. Are our beings saturated by these qualities, or are our surfaces just scratched by them?

The qualities chosen here for review are not all the qualities of being that exist. It is up to each of us to discover or invent those qualities we find important to creating a healthy vital life. Of course, feel free to make them up—to imagine whatever you would like. Once imagined, bring them into full manifestation in your life.

And a word about each quality. There is a common theme among them. How do they feel to you? How do they register with you when examined? What does your soul say to you when asked about them? You see, you can read a good book, enjoy the story, enjoy the drama, but are you able to put yourself into the story and notice the impact of events on your Self?

This is the possibility before you—to uncover an amazing life— by embracing these qualities and then living them. I don't know the outcome, but I can imagine it. It is up to each of us how we live life with these qualities that I state are essential to good health— something else I simply made up . . . and perhaps lived a bit too :).

You get to decide for yourself. And you get to see whether you become healthier or not, whether you are experiencing life with greater vitality, joyfulness, enthusiasm, sense of adventure, playfulness, fun, or not. Are you in love with life? Are you in love with your Self?

• • •

Chapter 18
BEING

The word *qualities* is familiar to most of us. The word *Being* deserves further description and explanation as we examine together the qualities of being. The state of being, or beingness, is what is in this moment.

Even the last moment, isn't anymore. And the future one doesn't exist yet. Neither are in being. Only *NOW* is in a state of beingness. So, to bring yourself into being, bring yourself into the Now moment. That is all there is to it. And to keep this simple—always my intention whenever possible—become comfortable with just allowing that the now moment is all there is for each of us. And everyone's now moment is different for each of us too.

To reflect upon yesterday, we are present to a memory of an experience that no longer is. To reflect upon that which we will do tomorrow is reflecting upon a moment that for us, isn't, also—not unless you are consciously engaged in the process of dreaming your life into being. That's a different realm, a different dimension, and a valid one. Dreaming will be one of the chapters in this part. We will get to consider that something can be and not be at the same time.

This first chapter of Part II is *Being* because I think it is a great starting point for the ideas expressed here—to literally *be with* all that is presented and to *be with it in the Now moment* . . . this ups the ante on your presence in your own life's creation.

Nothing else to say about this experience except, enjoy the journey!

Chapter 19
LOVE

"You, yourself, as much as anybody in the entire universe,
deserve your love and affection."

Buddha

I would like you all to know that I had nothing to do with the selection of the title of this next chapter. As I mentioned in the beginning that I believe Love is itself intelligent. So, *Love* just pushed itself into the front of the line, desiring to be talked about next. As I reflected upon this, I realize that perhaps Love is at the foundation of everything. It seems to be that way for me, maybe or maybe not for you.

To bring this thought home to you in a more meaningful way, just consider anything that (or who) we ever loved before, suddenly disappearing. How does (did) that change our life and the living of it? We have all lost something or someone we have loved, sometimes over and over again. This can be the source of much sadness, grief, sense of loss.

For some of us, looking back later we can appreciate how that love and that experience enhanced and enriched our life. (For the record I would like to acknowledge that I have not written a word of what was just stated. Love did. All this just came through and my fingers on this keyboard put them into words).

I believe Love is present throughout the universe, is present in All there is. It could be that love is experienced differently here on earth than elsewhere—maybe because most of us don't experience unconditional love here yet. I think the world would look and feel much different it we did.

I believe it is important to distinguish what Love is—like we distinguished between the lower self and the Higher Self in the beginning of our journey together. I could talk about the lower love and the Higher Love with you in the same way, but I won't. I will leave it up to each of you to figure out. You are all becoming (or have been all along) very smart in this area of uncovering Truth. So please, let each of us look at the many ways we think of what love with a little 'l' represents, and what Love with a large 'L' represents. Let's all reflect upon this before proceeding to the next paragraph.

I have been in love a number of times . . . or so I thought! Yes, I can feel you snickering now. And I know some of you are even laughing at me, with me, and perhaps even at yourselves. Most of us have been here before. What have we learned about love having traversed these magical waters with all the unseen dangers of the deep present but not realized until later? And where did it bring us? This then is the heart of this chapter, no pun intended.

Love appears at the beginning of Part II because—aside from its insistence to be at the beginning—it may facilitate the digestion of all that is to follow with an air of acceptance of oneself in the light of love. Perhaps Love's sister, Forgiveness, will show herself, will teach us the importance of forgiving our Selves and others as we explore and deepen our experience of this quality called *Love*—of little 'l' and Large 'L'.

A long time ago I was sitting in the front row of a course being presented by Louise Hay on Self-Healing in Boston. She passed around a mirror to those of us in the front row and asked us to look at ourselves in it, and then state while looking at our own image, "I love you." I couldn't do it. At the time I realized I didn't love myself. And I got to look at why not?!

I then spent the rest of my life discovering the importance of this one quality, this quality of loving oneself. For me it meant far more than just saying the words, it meant meaning them at every level of my being, and within every cell of my body. It amounts to total acceptance of oneself at all levels of life and living. How do you know when one truly loves oneself? Stay tuned! That's where this chapter is going.

And now, just for the fun of it I am going to cut to the chase and deliver the punch line before the story goes further. Then we will develop this thought together and how to perhaps arrive at this awareness.

You see, I have discovered that we must first love ourselves unconditionally before we can genuinely love others or be loved by them. And of course, this is not an original thought with me. It has been said in many of the ancient words of others and ancient writings of many cultures. But these are just more words until we do the work, until we discover them within our own beings, embrace and embody them as our own experience. Then the journey begins in a whole new light.

Many of us may have experienced love with a little 'l' like romantic love. We fall in love easily and a while later something changes, and we are not in love anymore. Perhaps love is the wrong word for this. Perhaps we need to invent a new one. In the Q'uechuan language of the Q'ero of Peru, *munay* means unconditional love. *Hatun munay* means greatest unconditional love. Or we can distinguish love with a small 'l' and a large 'L'. Make something up that creates a more accurate distinction for you.

I believe that romantic love can also be love with a large 'L'. Partner-love, parent- child love, love of a creation we are responsible for, love of a place or experience, can all be spelled with a small 'l' or a large 'L'. It depends entirely upon who we are and how we are showing up in life. I am only suggesting here that if we show up as unconditionally loving our Selves, we then can give and receive love unconditionally—without stipulations, rules, requirements, etc. etc. that is to say, all the things we humans come up with to thwart genuine heartfelt experiences.

I now see all these rules of engagement, these stipulations we humans are constantly imposing upon each other, as nothing more than a need to control and dominate others, and they grow out of fear and a lack of love—a lack of Self-love specifically. And don't allow your ego a vote on this. We all experience this. We are all perpetrators of this need to control and dominate until we see what is going on and we stop it. We are also all victims of it too, until we discover we do not need to be, and stop it.

I guess since we are on the triangle that my Shaman's Altar training brought to my awareness, I will complete it by mentioning the 3rd side of the triangle, that of the rescuer. In essence we each show up at various times as one of the three—as Perpetrator, Victim, or Rescuer. The important thing is to perhaps first notice we are on the triangle. The next important thing is to consciously get off of it. Stay with me please. This is all bringing us to an awareness of Selflove, of unconditional Selflove. And this you will want for the rest of your lives. Trust me, but don't believe a word I say until you try it on for yourself :)

To be sure we are all on the same page, allow me to remind each of us that unconditional means no conditions, no reasons to have or not, *no thing* other than the quality of love, which is a quality of its beingness, its isness, in this very moment and none other. Love simply IS. And it may be at the heart of creation.

As you all know and are now aware of, I wish to keep things simple and straightforward. This is true for Love too. Let's look together at Love simply.

Some of you may be rolling your eyes again, saying that love is possibly one of the most complicated experiences of life and living, a topic fraught with sadness, grief, loss, when it isn't experienced the other way many of us have also known it—with a sense of great joy, exciting and thrilling, unimaginable happiness, and yes, our hearts feeling deeply touched . . . until it goes away. Where does it go? I can't speak for anyone else but have heard time and time again how love was lost by someone. I've experienced this too, over and over again. Does anyone know what I'm talking about? How many people have had their hearts broken over lost love?

I will assert something radical now, and it will be simple. This will require every one of us to accept love with the large 'L', just like I suggested we listen to our Higher Self—with the big 'S'—instead of the self with the little 's'. We've all learned that distinction now, or at least been exposed to it in an earlier chapter. This may still be marinating for some of us, but consider it has merit in providing us eventually with great health and happiness. Just a point of view but something to consider.

You see, when we are able to love our SELF unconditionally— Hatun Munay—the rest becomes easy. It is getting to loving one's SELF that presents difficulty for some of us until we simply begin loving our SELF. Then it becomes easy and simple.

For some of us, we have already discovered the formula. If you haven't, ask your SELF what it would take for you to unconditionally love your SELF? You could list a bunch of qualities you would first need to acquire or possess or embody to love yourself this way. This may work but may also be a never-ending list in which you will love yourself when the list is complete, and the list never becomes complete. It's the *Someday, One Day* experience we've all known. *Someday* never arrives.

Until we say it does. Until we say we are complete. This is an act of power, of SELF empowerment. And no one is going to bestow it upon us. We get to do that for ourselves. It's an honor and a privilege. And it's totally up to each of us to decide when we reached this level of Love. You'll know.

I mentioned earlier that I had the opportunity to look into a mirror and say to my SELF, *I love you*, but I couldn't. I can now. I don't recall when this happened. It's not like I was looking into a mirror every day and finally discovered one day I loved myself. It just eventually happened.

Perhaps at the core of this was this notion of forgiveness. I had to forgive myself for all my transgressions, for all the things that I considered causing harm to another, for all thoughts and deeds that I considered were not of kindness, compassion, or of this higher love. And I discovered that all those things are qualities we all perhaps may have experienced in one form or another, to a greater or lesser degree. They are all qualities of being human. And it's up to each of us to decide and say *no more* to the things we don't like, the things we don't wish to participate in anymore. It comes down to individual choice again. Little by little we begin to notice how we are showing up in the world and we begin to like it. And little by little the world shows up differently to us, and we begin to like it. And it will be different for every one of us because we are all unique beings.

At some point, each of us will be able to look into a mirror and say, *I love you*. And then we will know that loving unconditionally has arrived. Thank you, Louise Hay!

There will be many opportunities to test each of us. For some of us it will not be a matter of only forgiving ourselves but forgiving others who may have harmed or hurt us, some who may not deserve our forgiveness given the extent of the harm they have caused. Many of us have our stories.

History is full of stories of terrible suffering and abuse at the hands of others. It is up to us to decide where we wish to weigh in on this decision, this act of forgiveness or not. Many of us have heard stories and witnessed events where forgiveness was rendered and it changed the lives of the person forgiving, and the one(s) being forgiven. But the point is, this is for you, and your SELF, on your path to unconditional love and comprehensive healing on all levels. Just another opinion and one that each of us will act upon or not, discover what may lie beyond or not. Do you wish to remain part of a story you don't like? If not, rewrite it then. You've already learned how to do this.

Just remember, there is no *I love you because* . . . There is only, *I love*. There are no reasons to love. It is a state of being, a state of love, no conditions imposed.

This is unconditional love. This is *Hatun Munay*. This is possible for all of us. And this will make the greatest difference in our lives. This will make all the difference in a world so in need of unconditional love.

That was simple, was it not? Now let's get to it. How and where will you begin?

"You, yourself, as much as anybody in the entire universe, deserve your love and affection."

Buddha

Chapter 20
FORGIVENESS

"If we really want to love we must learn how to forgive."
Mother Teresa

This is very interesting. You just heard me tell you in Chapter 19 how Love just pushed its way to the front of the line to start that chapter. Well, the same just happened with Forgiveness. We've already talked of Forgiveness being Love's sister, perhaps the simple reason it demanded to be included now right after Love. You know how family can be sometimes! Let us just surrender to the possibility that perhaps this is the perfect place to discuss Forgiveness, forgiving oneself, forgiving others.

I suspect we'll discover this quality—forgiveness—is very important to all the other qualities of being we will talk about, and essential to achieving great health. It could be that without owning this one quality all the others don't completely get the job done. Let's examine it together now. And please don't get too attached to what I say. There may be some tough spots here for some of us, maybe for most of us. Remember, I am making it all up . . . until you try it on for yourself and decide its merit, or not. I am not making up the parts where I quote others. Those thoughts can be viewed as their gift to you. Maybe some more value here . . . just maybe:)

There is another quote that reflects the untarnished innocence of early childhood: *"Every adult was once a child free from prejudice."*

141

If you guessed Mother Teresa as the source, you were right. She had a lot to say about Forgiveness and lived her life out of what many would say was out of pure Love.

If you recall in the early part of this book, I suggested seeing the world through the eyes of a child before that child is altered by the realities of the world we know, the world of consensual reality where that child's view is now altered and perhaps contaminated and corrupted by forces outside itself. That world of the early child can be called the bliss state. We each have it when we are born into it, then lose it, then spend most of our lives searching for it.

Let's digress for a moment for an anatomy lesson, specifically, the anatomy of forgiveness. As a surgeon I am familiar with anatomy of a physical nature. I am a novice at the anatomy of forgiveness. In fact, this is the first time I considered writing about it but thought it may be useful to look at it together. This could be even more difficult than surgery.

A common dictionary definition for what it means *to forgive: to let go of anger, blame or resentment towards someone and return to friendly relations.*

Perhaps we have all experienced some variations of these emotions—anger, blame, resentment towards another, and likely towards ourselves at times. What happened to cause these emotions of anger, blame, resentment to arise within us? What was the injury, the insult, the transgression, that caused them to arise in the first place? Pay attention! We may get our lives out of this conversation.

I would suggest that there is a distinction between *letting go* and *a return to friendly relations,* the latter perhaps being more difficult than the former. We may all be able to agree that small insults and injuries are easier to let go of than big ones. Why is that? The size of the wound matters to some of us, maybe most of us.

This conversation is going to lead us into some uncharted waters—one of my nautical terms—because it may be unfamiliar or unknown to many of us. And in the interest of becoming truly healthy, I am going to suggest that enormous leaps of faith may be called for. Just remember, this is all for the best life we can imagine. I have nothing to sell you. They are all just words and ideas to consider and work with in the grand laboratory called *Life*.

What would it take for us to forgive something that happened to us, something we could let go of and move on? I'll suggest we have all been here before. And then what about those things that are totally unforgiveable? Many of us have experienced our share of these things too to a greater or lesser degree—all on a continuum from *not so bad to horrible and unimaginable*. Each of us can draw our own lines of tolerance or not.

First, I want to inform you all that I am going for nothing less than extraordinary in our lives in all things . . . *ALL THINGS*. Much will be easy (effortless ease), some not so easy, some very difficult, but all with the same prize in sight. Each of us gets to choose for ourselves. Doing nothing is fine too.

I began this section (Part II) with Being, Love, and Forgiveness, perhaps the most difficult qualities and topics we humans can grapple with in our lives. Since this book is dedicated to our health, and the art of creating it, and the fiction that may be utilized as we create it, I am hopeful some of these words have an impact on your lives. Since I have studied health most of my adult life, and since I maintain integrity and honesty in my intentions and deeds, some of you will agree that I have your best interests in mind and in heart.

Few topics generate more emotion than the memories of sustaining pain and suffering at the hands of another, and even more so, at the act of forgiving those for the serious wounds inflicted. And yet, this is exactly what I am going to suggest—in degrees, in shades of gray, in small bits only as one can tolerate. We each have different degrees of tolerance. I believe this is an ultimate path to healing, so I am sharing it with you. You do not need to agree or follow this path. Perhaps consider it though.

For those of us who are fortunate enough to have loved ones in our sphere, we have probably discovered that that support in our lives is invaluable. Not all of us have this. What other forms of support have we turned to for the really difficult issues in our lives? This is a good time to make a list of what you see. It will be useful later if not now. If you see nothing, that's useful too.

Now for a practice session: Pick the littlest thing that happened to you for which you found it easy to forgive—not to forget, but to forgive. Keep a record. Now pick one that you feel you could never forgive no matter what. Sorry for dredging up old or unpleasant memories whether recent or remote, but to a purpose—and just a practice session, remember. Now pick one somewhere in the middle, difficult to forgive, but doable and you have done it after consideration. Notice these all live on a spectrum of past events.

If they are current and happening to you now, things which require your forgiveness, it is time to bring an end to it. Talk about it, state your feelings, draw a line in the sand, and move on. Let go of the perpetrator, the person, the job, the afflicting entity. Get free from it. It is not how humans were designed to live.

Notice how the minor ones were easier to forgive. Notice the transition zone, where maybe forgiveness was possible even though not comfortable forgiving. And then, those acts you judged were just not forgivable. Look at what if would take to move those unforgivable acts perpetrated on you into the possibly forgivable zone, then perhaps to move them further into the forgivable zone. Who would you have to become to generate complete forgiveness for anyone or anything for an unspeakable act committed against you, one that harmed you mentally, emotionally, or physically, even wounded your soul?

For this exercise, look at yourself in the moment, in this NOW moment. What is so for you right now? Is this the story you want to carry through life? Whatever your affliction or disability—mental, emotional, or physical—do you see further healing is possible? I will assert that further healing is always possible. Let's look together at what this may take. No matter how difficult, my intention is to keep this as simple as possible for us, to make it as accessible to us as possible and perhaps lead to an extraordinary life ahead for each of us.

There is a trust piece here. You are aware that I have spent most of my adult life studying health and what it takes to be very healthy. I know I've said before, "Don't trust a word I say." Try it on first, consider it, put it to the test in your own life first, then decide its merit, or not. So, the trust I am suggesting here is simply to accept that I have your own best interests at heart, which is the same as having my own best (self) interests at heart too. We're in this together, remember?

I am not the first or only person to suggest that forgiveness is a path to healing. Many others have and have found healing. Those forgiven have also found healing. I have been in this place before and have experienced healing in forgiveness. There is no question of this for me anymore. I would like you to simply consider this, perhaps discover this for yourself. School is still out as to whether total comprehensive healing is possible in the absence of being able to forgive. My early guess is that it is not. Like there is no such thing as a bit of unconditional love. It is either unconditional love or not. What do you think?

In this section that may present some difficulty in degrees of forgiveness, complete forgiveness, or none, I will rely on the words of others I respect, some of whom have much more experience in the art of forgiveness. Hence, the following quotes. Note that I just researched these quotes so new to me too, and I feel worth sharing.

ON FORGIVENESS

Forgiveness says you are given another chance to make a new beginning.

--Desmond Tutu

There is no love without forgiveness, and there is no forgiveness without love

--Bryant H. McGill

Forgiveness is the fragrance that the violet sheds on the heel that has crushed it.

--Mark Twain

145

To forgive is to set a prisoner free and discover that the prisoner was you.

--Lewis B. Smedes.

All major religious traditions carry basically the same message; that is love, compassion and forgiveness. The important thing is they should be part of our daily lives.

--Dalai Lama

I think the first step is to understand that forgiveness does not exonerate the perpetrator. Forgiveness liberates the victim. It is a gift you give yourself.

--T D Jakes

You can't forgive without loving. And I don't mean sentimentality. I don't mean mush. I mean having the courage to stand up and say, 'I forgive. I'm finished with it.'

--Maya Angelou

It's not an easy journey, to get to a place where you forgive people. But it is such a powerful place, because it frees you.

--Tyler Perry

How unhappy is he who cannot forgive himself.

--Publilius Syrus

Forgiveness is giving up the hope that what would have, could have, should have happened, in fact . . . it did not happen. It's accepting the reality of what did happen, and moving on . . . This truth has been fundamental in allowing me to live my best life. It was transformative. You have to come to the realization that what might have been is not what is.

--Oprah

We must develop and maintain the capacity to forgive. He who is devoid of the power to forgive is devoid of the power to love.

--Martin Luther King Jr

It is one of the greatest gifts you can give yourself, to forgive. Forgive everybody.

--Maya Angelou

True forgiveness is when you can say, thank you for that experience.

--Oprah

Take forgiveness slowly. Don't blame yourself for being slow. Peace will come.

--Yoko Ono

Forgiveness is healing—especially forgiving yourself.

--Alyson Noel

Forgiveness does not mean ignoring what has been done or putting a false label on an evil act. It means, rather, that the evil act no longer remains as a barrier to the relationship. Forgiveness is a catalyst creating the atmosphere necessary for a fresh start and a new beginning.

--Martin Luther King Jr

Forgiveness is not weak. It takes courage to face and overcome powerful emotions.

--Desmond Tutu Nobel Peace Prize laureate

Mistakes are always forgivable if one has the courage to admit them.

--Bruce Lee

As I walked out the door toward the gate that would lead me to my freedom, I knew if I didn't leave my bitterness and hated behind, I'd still be in prison.

--Nelson Mandela

Let's shake free this gravity of judgment / And fly high on the wings of forgiveness.

--India Arie

I believe forgiveness is the best form of love in any relationship. It takes a strong person to say they're sorry and an even stronger person to forgive.

--Yolanda Hadid

If one by one we counted people out / For the least sin, it wouldn't take us long / To get so we had no one left to live with. / For to be social is to be forgiving.

--Robert Frost

Love deeper / Speak sweeter / Give forgiveness

--Gigi Hadid

The only way out of the labyrinth of suffering is to forgive.

--John Green

When someone wrongs you, you don't forgive them for them, you forgive them for you.

--Christine Lakin

Forgiveness is designed to set you free. When you say, I forgive you, what you're really saying is I know what you did is not okay, but I recognize that you are more than that. I don't want to hold us captive to this thing anymore. I can heal myself, and I don't need anything from you.

--Sarah Montana (from a TED talk)

(Sarah lost her family due to gun violence by the hand of a friend of her brother's who pulled the trigger).

If it appears that I stacked the deck in favor of us all recognizing the importance of forgiveness in our lives, you are right. I did. I did this for myself too. I know that I wanted to be complete in forgiving myself and everyone in my life that I felt I needed to forgive. This made a difference. I've had a sense for a long time that forgiveness was important for healing in our lives.

The act of forgiving is such a charged issue however that not until I began writing a chapter on it did it cause me to look into it deeper and discover what others had to say about it. The list of quotes above is only a fraction of what is said about forgiveness. I included enough of them so there may be something to inspire each of us to at least consider it.

Feel free to search the many quotes available and find some that call to you. Feel free to write your own if you can summon up the courage to walk the path of forgiveness for yourself and for others. And if you commit to this path, remember it is not just rendering lip service to forgiving and hoping it slips by. Forgiveness needs to be experienced by every cell in your body and especially your whole heart, i.e. experienced wholeheartedly. I'm just making this up, but it feels right. You decide for yourself.

Remember also, this is all for you. You can think of anything left unforgiven for you is like leaving a chain or a shackle attached to your body holding you back from the fullest life you can imagine.

And there may be a payoff for the ones forgiven too but that's another realm and will be deferred for later. Recall that I have stated that everything is connected. There are no secrets in the unseen realms.

Chapter 21
FAMILY

Good topic! Interesting how it just showed up following Love and Forgiveness. For some of us this could also present as a difficult chapter—read that as a difficult childhood as perceived by some of us (including me), or a difficult adulthood as perceived by some of us (including me), or anywhere on the map—and for some of us this may be an area where great joy and gratitude show up for us. I was part of the former group until I dug deep enough to see the hidden gifts. I then shifted. I now have much gratitude for all the life lessons I learned from family—the good, the bad, and the ugly.

Some of you may have noticed that Part II is titled *Qualities of Being*, and some may be wondering if Forgiveness or Family are qualities. This is where I assert writer's prerogative in making things up. Consider that each chapter presented in Part II may have a great deal to do with affecting our lives when each is considered in depth, and specifically, perhaps very much affecting the quality of our lives. That is my intention. Enough said.

A few years ago, I got the notion that I would shift my focus from what it takes to create comprehensive health for an individual to what it would take to create a healthy family, one that is based on shared love and joy and truly is well in all domains of family, one in which each member is there for each other in all ways regardless of circumstance. *That can be read as unconditionally there for each other no matter what.* Does that expression ring a bell for a few of you?

Some of you already experience this—that family love and cohesiveness are present for you and shared by you and your family in a healthy wholehearted way. From my actual experience in the world of HealthCare, I can say that many of us do not share this experience. We will look at this *phenomenon* together and see how a healthy family may contribute to greater health, happiness, contentment, wellbeing. Maybe another tough journey for some of us, but one which I feel is worth taking. And I'll be on this journey with you too. Could this be another Bilbo Baggins adventure? You decide.

I chose to look at this area when I began looking closer at what more could I say about becoming healthy. It occurred to me, that there is much about family life that presents as difficult for its members, over generations, over continents. I began to wonder what the world would look like if all family members got along with each other within their family . . . always. And then this expanded to my wondering what the world would look like if all families got along with every other family. I hear some of you laughing already but consider that every dream begins somewhere.

My daughter, Paige, gave me a hollow wooden triangular-shaped piece of artwork for Christmas last year which had a light on the inside. The block letters carved into it reads, *DREAM BIG.* The light within would illuminate the letters in the dark. It now always sits on a prominent counter in my home as a daily reminder. It is also the title of a poem I wrote several years ago. I believe in it. I believe Dreams are important to us. Dreaming will be a chapter in this book as I mentioned earlier. Stay tuned if you want to learn more on dream magic.

Now back on track to wondering about what the world would look like if all families got along with each other in each family, and then imagining if all families got along with all other families. Sounds like a dream world to me. Consider that if you can imagine something, that you can create it. To really sound far-reaching right now, consider that

151

if you've thought of it, it already exists somewhere in the future. Spooky thought, eh?

Let's take this in small bites. We are talking about big things here. But remember, you have already signed up for the advanced course by picking up this book, particularly since you have gotten this far in the reading of it. I would like to suggest that nothing shocks you anymore from this point on, and I would like to invite you into a minor conspiracy—without all the baggage that word implies—by suggesting that perhaps you and I can change the world for the better.

Remember that stone thrown into the pond of life creating ripples that spread outward throughout the universe endlessly? This is one of those. Just thinking this can make a difference without doing anything else. Taking it to the next level— perhaps we begin mentioning this to others in our own words, writing about it, creating a poem or a song or a piece of art or a story or a movie, whatever our form of self-expression is—will help manifest the world we desire to live in. Let's see what shows up. And once you create something like this you get to talk about it with others, describe it, engage them in dream making of their own. You might notice, I am already doing this. I've accepted the challenge. Join me, anyone?

Does anyone recall reading The Hundredth Monkey by Kenneth Keyes? It is an interesting true story. I will summarize since it is pertinent to our conversation about changing the world.

A monkey on a particular island off Japan was observed to be going to the ocean to wash a sweet potato. This recurred with some frequency, and eventually the observers started noting other monkeys coming to the ocean to wash their potatoes. About the time they counted 100 monkeys washing their potatoes on that island, it was later noted that monkeys on other islands began doing the same thing. Neither population had any observed contact with the monkeys on the other islands, yet that same activity became a common practice and eventually spread even further. You have to read the book for more details. I read it many years ago.

The point of the story was that about the time a behavior increases to a small percentage of the population, behaviors are then transmitted

152

to other parts of the world even when there has been no visible contact. Moral of the story—It only takes a few of the total number of any population to alter behaviors, activities, etc.

Since then, I've heard a better one. It only takes two individuals totally aligned in thought, deed, action, and in Spirit, to change something in the world. I'll just mention this to pique your curiosity to investigate further. There are more stories, but for God's sake don't trust me! Explore this. I'm a scientist. Apply the scientific principle to your research. Let me know what you discover. The 100th Monkey is worth the read too. I just searched it and got an instant summary of the work.

Now, anyone interested in changing the world with their thoughts, activities, deeds, intentions, etc.? It won't take many of us :)

We haven't deviated too far. Talking about a family of monkeys isn't too much different than talking about a family of humans. I'll offer no further comparative comments on this subject.

I will however continue the conversation, and given my inclination to spontaneity and innovation, I must mention last night. I was invited to an evening movie on the North Shore of my island (Kaua'i), attended by about 30 others. It was a documentary called *Terrain* and the Director was in attendance to discuss and answer questions. The movie has not been released to the public yet via theaters or online links. This was the first public showing as the Director stated. It is worth seeing and it was revealing as to the state of the world. It was well researched. I will not talk about it. You can watch it and form your own opinions.

What did catch my attention, and something I want to share, was a segment on the work of Veda Austin on *The Secret Intelligence of Water*. She is a New Zealander and has been engaged in this research for years, as have others. What is clearly revealed in her work, in addition to her passion, is that water is conscious, has intelligence, and willingly communicates with us humans—and probably all forms of life. This goes a few notches beyond the 100th Monkey story. I won't say more about it now but suggest it may be an important pathway to

153

healing. Research it for yourself and see what you find. I will suggest it is well worth it. And I feel it belongs in this chapter on Family.

What I have stated before is that we are all connected to each other and to everything. The more I look and experience, the more this notion is reaffirmed for me. This could be a grand description of Family. Happy to hear your thoughts on this exploration and possibility. I will include some of these in my next book if there are any responses. This is a shared community experience, and all our reflections matter. Maybe this can be called a shared Family experience.

Let's shift gears into a more concerning aspect of family life, that of the cause or contribution to dis-ease states. In my role as a physician, I have encountered considerable pathology that arose out of family experiences, as shared with me over years by various family members in a wide variety of clinical settings. Stories of pain and suffering, injury and abuse, within family units are as astonishing as they are common. I also studied family and learned about family through the writings of others, the courses I took, and my own experience of family. So many stories.

I will suggest again something radical for each of us, in the interest of the pursuit of extraordinary health. It may align with some comments in the chapter on Forgiveness. Actually, they may be intricately related.

We can look at this through the window of our mental emotional composition, the health of our personal constitutions, our experiences here on planet Earth from a hereditary or environmental perspective, or from a karmic or spiritual perspective, not to mention the ancestorial imprints that I discussed earlier in this book. This is a lot to consider and sounds complex.

Perhaps an exercise: List your family concerns, illnesses, experiences that you feel contributed to disease states, or stress, which is also linked to disease states as we noted earlier. Keep it simple, because the list can become long, even overwhelming, but worth noting just for a deeper look at how this shows up in your family, and in your own life. Whether it is cancer, or heart disease, inflammatory bowel disease, or any other system in our bodies, it is important to notice how extensively our health and wellbeing are affected by many things. There are so many dis-ease states. Just scan through a Harrison's Textbook of Medicine for a glimpse. And the list is ever-expanding, as are the number of medications manufactured to address these conditions. Maybe another approach is more useful.

Rather than throwing the baby out with the bath water—meaning keep the good stuff, get rid of the bad—what if we just drop it all, all the notions that any of the old junk plays a role anymore? Design a new story out of the new paradigm, and simply move forward as a better human being. What is a better human being? We already discussed this in earlier chapters. What would it take to become one? We discussed that before too. Reread the material if you forgot them or are confused. Most important is you get to decide *for you*. Try it on. Improvise and create uninhibitedly. How does it feel in your body?

Of course, generating qualities like love and forgiveness and kindness and compassion may be of value, along with the importance of cleaning house. Empty it all out! No dust left in the corners, nothing that doesn't serve you anymore— nothing that doesn't serve your family, or friends, or neighbors, or community, either. Just look! It's all there. You just must see if it is worth keeping or not. What kind of a world do you want to create? Would you like the world's population to learn how to wash their potatoes—maybe their lives too—in the ocean of life? I believe cleaner is better. What do you believe?

And don't forget, this catches on quickly, like in the 100th Monkey, like how quickly water can recreate an image of an object or a thought in its proximity. Is anyone willing to play? :)

Before we leave this chapter, I want to be sure we've explored all the dark places in our lives so we can be complete in cleaning them out. Listen, we are talking about nothing less than the transformation of humanity as we've known it, and I would suggest we start NOW, and be done NOW, with the process. Just say YES to this quantum leap. It's like going from point A to point B without traversing the space in between—a quantum leap in another dimension, but one available to each of us when we tune into it. Anybody want to ante up, throw their chips into the center of the table and join the game?

You see, I believe we have all arrived at a high stakes game. The quality of our lives is at stake. Life itself as we would like to experience it in our dream world is clearly at stake. I assert this is intricately related to Family. If you and I believe in the creation of a healthy happy family of this nature, of families like this everywhere in our world, then it is worth everything we can each bring to the table in this moment, and then we simply continue to bring it. Yes, for always.

Look now into your own family, how you have lived it, how you are living it now, and what are you willing to do to make it a better experience for all. And what are you willing to offer your community? What are you willing to offer the world? Consider this is only an expansion of a Family of which you are already a part.

And while you're looking, take an extra few moments to create your dream experience of family for you, and for how you would like to see all families living and being together. And for God's sake, get comfortable with dreaming! You should be getting good at this by now. You've had lots of experience at creating your own design for anything. Try it out on Family now. What did you come up with? Are you already living your dream? If not, what's missing?

Now what?

Speaking of Family and before we leave this chapter, I will mention that I invited my son, John, to share any thoughts he had with the world just like the invitation went out to the Goddesses appearing in Part III. And like the Goddesses, there were no rules on length, no editing, just whatever was there to say. This is what he had to say . . .

SHARED THOUGHTS FROM MY SON

"So recently my father asked me to write a contribution to his book, his first book ever, this book, and I thought what an honor. As I started thinking about what I wanted to write, I would start overthinking what I wanted to be immortalized on pages in a book forever. This caused me to procrastinate and keep putting off my writing. It was discussed in a family video chat to just write whatever came to my mind, no pressure, no certain points to hit, and just let it flow from the heart. This eased my tension about writing, and I sat down and started letting my fingers do the work that my mind couldn't before. I realized how easy it is to get in my own way sometimes, and that all you really need to do sometimes, is just speak or write truly, from the heart, and with conviction. I really enjoyed that video call.

"So, I am the only son, born into a family of 4 sisters, my mom and dad. I am 26 years old, one month from being 27. To me, my family is one of the most important aspects in my life, and always has been. The bond I have with them is something I wouldn't trade for anything. The word family, to me, means trust, it means being there for each other, it means unconditional love, among so many other things. My family is also my blood, although it doesn't have to be. It just must be people you love and trust and can totally be yourself around. I realize that some people don't get to experience what it feels like to belong to such a group of people, which is why I really cherish and am forever grateful for the one I was born into. It's a sacred bond that cannot be broken, and that requires a level of respect unmatched by most other things in life.

"There have certainly been ups and downs in my family life and life in general, and I haven't always treated my family with the respect they deserved. But they loved me when I couldn't love myself. I've had social struggles, physical struggles when I was a kid, and even struggles with addiction, and throughout everything, my family has always been by my side. There's been really amazing times, and really hard, difficult times, and I wouldn't go back and change a thing. Everything that's happened has brought me to this moment in time and made me the person I am today, and I love who I am today and who I'm becoming. I'm so very blessed to have such an amazing and wonderful family I can always rely on. My Dad is such an amazing father figure in my life and someone I really look up to. I have huge shoes to fill. I'll conclude my part by restating how much of an honor it is to be included in this book. Love you dad."

Chapter 22
LISTEN TO THE CHILDREN

Yes, children are part of Family and I also felt they deserved their own chapter, a special focus on this stage of life. You see, I think Children are a National Treasure... for all Nations. It is a state all of us human beings get to pass through if we survive it. Many don't.

You might notice there is a flavor of seriousness to these recent chapters—light and playful at times, but deadly serious at times too. Serious, like we are talking about not only the health and wellbeing of every human being on this planet, but also recognizing it is time to act on what it takes to create this ideal. Currently we are not being very successful at it . . . my opinion.

Serious, like we are talking about the health and survival of our very home called Earth, or more accurately and affectionately, *Mother Earth*. It helps to add *Mother* to Earth as it makes her more personal to us. She is indeed a being who is supporting us while we are here, in all kinds of ways. You don't need to think of her this way but many cultures close to her do. Your choice again, like in everything else. It may even be useful to think of all of us as children of Mother Earth.

If you've ever seen a hurt or sad or hungry child many of you know what that stirs within you. If you've caused it, change that behavior now. I won't speak of shame or guilt, but both are to be let go of. They do not serve us. And this is not to lay blame on anyone for cruel and heartless acts of aggression or violence that has caused immeasurable pain and suffering in the world, because many of us only knew this from being *taught it*—read that as experienced it—as children ourselves.

The point of even taking this approach in the beginning of this chapter on children is to give us all the opportunity to see something different perhaps in a way that assists us in changing our ways if they need changing. Again, no judgment on good or bad experiences here, just experiences—just an opportunity to look deeper and create better, healthier, maybe more joyful, experiences from here on. I will suggest this could contribute to a better world for all of us, not to mention serve to make us healthier as individuals. See this then as an opportunity for change. You see, it must begin somewhere and sometime. Why not *WITH YOU* and *NOW*?

As an observation of what is so in the world today, we could do better for our children. After we bring them into the world many are simply ignored, mistreated, abused, or discarded. Many aren't too. Since I'm aiming for 100%, I will just offer up some thoughts on what I sense our children want.

For starters, look back at what you wanted as a child. What was missing for you? If nothing, great! If something, look at it. See it. Feel it. Notice if you've carried it forward into your adult life and still feel something is missing. Notice if you are conveying this same thing that's missing for you to your own children if you have any. And feel no guilt or shame about it. Just become aware and grow from it.

Something I've observed over my life is that much of life is lived out of fear rather than love, out of the need to control and dominate, rather than communicate and relate in a mutually agreeable way. What would it take to make this a universal experience? Remember the 100th Monkey? We don't need many of us, but I still recommend 100% of us do this, kind of like a security blanket. We all win.

As an adult with children (or one without any), we add the responsibility of not only managing our own lives but of being effective at relating to all children. Guiding them into their preteen years and then into teenage years, arriving at young adulthood, is an awesome job, requires great skill, and calls for our very best within each of us. I don't expect any of us to change to be like this in a heartbeat, but then again, why not?! Consider it. Become the change we'd like to see in the world.

Since this notion is new for some of us, take some time to consider it—like a week or two—and then begin acting on it. Just thinking about it is taking action. Actually doing something to back this notion up is even more definitive action.

What would that look like? Usually I let you all figure this out on your own by now since we have all become much more adept at this process. However, I will make a suggestion via an example to drive my point home. This is a very important area. Consider a child—your child even—making a request of you to which your answer is *No*. How can you say the *No* to your child so the result is a smile on his or her face, a sign of agreement that your *No* was understood and appreciated at some level, even if the language skills aren't there yet? It's like speaking with your heart. A new language for some of us perhaps. This may take some practice.

I have five children, so I have had lots of practice, lots of opportunities to communicate and relate in the best way I knew how at the time. It wasn't always pretty, graceful, or successful, but I've improved I believe. You'll have to ask my children for their opinions. For me, I couldn't have done it without them.

We parents have the responsibility of raising our children and this includes guiding them to the best of our abilities. Too often guidance shows up like a need to control and dominate--how It may have been for us as children. There may be a fine line here, like seeing your child climb a tree for the first time. Do you just yell at them, tell them to stop, tell them they are going to get hurt—instill fear in them—or do you interact with them in a way that makes it a better experience for them, one where they may unconsciously perceive your concern (and love) for them without scaring them to death?

For example, you may even position yourself under them as they start to climb, encouraging them to do it safely, guiding each reach for the branch overhead, each foot placement. If they fall, you are there.

This happened to one of my girls, Julie. She was adept at climbing at an early age. We were hiking on a mountain to pick blueberries. Her younger sister Paige was with us. Julie spotted a big maple and wanted to climb it. There was no hesitation in my allowing it. I watched her ascend quickly as I spotted for her below. She had a daypack on and wore it for the climb. Suddenly she cried out as she began to fall. I was ready. But I wasn't needed. The tree caught her! Her daypack hung up on one of the branches and she just hung there, all of us laughing at this adventure. No one hurt. Perhaps a much better experience for her than a scolding or telling her I never want her in a tree again.

And I can relate as an adult, as I've had more than one tree landing under the canopy of my parachute. I know the feeling of being stopped on my way through the branches by the tree.

And on that same climb to pick blueberries, we came to a small cliff at the top. My girls wanted to climb it. This time Paige participated. She was about 4 at the time. It was fingers and toes only, for most of it. I spotted. Suddenly I became very nervous for her, scrambled up behind her and spotted from next to and below her. She made it! So did I. She was smiling. I was grateful she made it and happy.

While this was not a high cliff—only about 12 feet above the base—it was mostly straight up and a challenge, and they wanted to do it. I saw my job as parent to successfully supervise the experience while keeping them safe. We practiced certain climbing principles, and it was overall a very enjoyable experience.

My point of this entire story is to illustrate there are many ways we parents can interact with our children in a myriad of circumstances. If you saw this as risky, you need not do it with your child. I perceived it as a safe adventure and a learning experience. I believe our children will pick up on our energy. That is what may make all the difference, what we as parents bring to the interaction. But remember, always try to leave each child with a smile on his or her face. Perhaps you'll even have one too. Can you imagine what you look like to your child when that isn't there?

This introduction was a warmup to a topic near and dear to my heart. I hold family as very close. I hold children even closer. As it has been stated before, children are the future of the world. It matters greatly how we relate to them as they grow, how we nurture and nourish their growth. When I look at the condition of the world, and the experience of many children, I believe we could be doing a better job. What kind of a world are we preparing for our children's children?

Years ago, I did a project with photographs and poems and writing that was part of a 6-month long course. I titled it, *Listen to the Children*. It is not like children have all the answers for a world run by adults, but they may have valuable input and deserve a say in how they see their own lives unfolding. The very least we adults can do is listen to them, even better to listen to them like what they have to say really matters (because it does).

I have just decided that a future book that I want to write will show images of children, their play, their stories when known. When the story is unknown, I will ask you the reader to make up a story for them just by looking at a photo. You can do this. Remember, we are all connected. And your perceptions will appear in a future book if you agree.

You may be noticing that I am gradually bringing you into the world of children, gently, by invitation. It is an area in which we all have experience—good, bad, or ugly, depending upon our perceptions and experience, but still experience.

How many of you recall times as a child you felt not seen or not heard? I'll answer for all of us. I believe we have all been there. I believe we have all been there as adults too. That's my point. It is almost a universal phenomenon. How did we feel when this was experienced? How would you design it differently if you had the power to do so? Pretend you have that power now, how will you do it differently from this moment on? By the way, you do have that power.

Where this is going is simple, that we all become more conscious at listening to others, and at really seeing them. Begin with children. They are easy and so forgiving of us adults. Then practice with adults, a more difficult group overall, just another opinion based solely on my own experience. See what shows up for you as you practice.

And practice is what I suggest for the rest of our lives. Getting it better and better every day, more authentic, more loving, more caring, more playful, more anything that makes the world a better place. Use your imagination. Be as creative as your Spirit calls to you. Let's begin now.

By the way, all my kids ran track. In that world, it was the starter's gun that got them off the line. You pick whatever gets you going! And remember, there are many spectators in life. Plan to be on the field. That's where the action is.

Thank you to those of you who have agreed to play. And remember, playing is natural for children and we adults can learn from them.

Chapter 23
LISTEN TO OUR PETS

This is a tongue-in-cheek follow up to the last chapter, but one I wish to report I am very serious about. I know I am speaking to a large audience who has pets, and I know many of you (if not all of you) speak to them. I will go out on a limb here and suggest that perhaps many of you listen to them too. Nothing is excluded here. Does this apply to you?

This includes the obvious dogs and cats members of the family but extends to birds, mice, hamsters, snakes, fish, etc.—whatever you call a pet that you have welcomed into your home. My kids had a pet rat once. He was always climbing around on my shoulder, and I liked his company. One of my classmates in med school had a pet tarantula. Are you getting the picture? No limitations.

This conversation will lead us all into deeper water to good purpose, my intention ultimately. We touched on this in the earlier chapters—our listening abilities. More practice here. Perhaps more Self-discovery here.

Listening to our pets calls us to listen with other than our ears. It is not about sound waves bouncing up against our tympanic membranes (eardrums), causing them to vibrate, which is then picked up and interpreted by our neurological system as sounds that are then converted to a language we understand, and one in which we communicate with each other. Fascinating system, isn't it?

How many of you listen to your pets and understand them? Do you acknowledge this Is a form of communication? This is no different than when I suggested earlier that you listen to that part of your body that is trying to tell you something. Some of you can relate to this form of communication. I suspect that many of you mothers experienced communication with your babies yet to be born while in utero. I'm a father and I communicated with my unborn children while they were being carried in utero by their mother.

What is really being discussed here is refining our listening skills. It may make it easier when we accept that everything is connected to everything else . . . and that we are in constant communication with everything we wish to be in communication with. It's like dialing into a radio station, different broadcasts available to each of us depending upon the band width we select, the vibrational frequency. And there is a special language we can learn to facilitate this. It's like listening to Higher Self versus lower self, already covered in the early chapters.

Now I will ask you to take another leap of faith and trust that this form of communication can be between us and *anything else.*

When I first offered my course on *Nature & You,* I asked how many people talked to their plants. Many did. Then I asked how many got responses. None did in that first program. At least not until after the outdoor exercise. Then some learned to communicate and did. They got responses that were meaningful to their lives.

What I wish to reintroduce you to is our ability to listen. All this takes is awareness and willingness to listen via other than through our auditory apparatus called our ears. Many of us have heard of listening with our hearts. This is an example of different listening. Now it becomes about practice and refining what we hear from whatever source we choose.

Recall the 100th Monkey story. What was being communicated to monkeys on other islands around the time that 100th monkey traveled to the ocean's edge to wash his or her potato? How were those other island monkeys listening to allow this potato washing to happen on the other islands?

This becomes a fun journey. The more we communicate with and listen for responses the better we get at it. Take a walk in Nature. Talk to the trees, the grass, the wind, the water, the butterflies, the bees, the birds, the animals, anything! Then listen. You'll get better at it with practice. By the way, our ancestors have done this for ages. The closer we become to Mother Earth and all her beings—and to Father Sun, Grandmother Moon, etc, as they are referred to in some cultures—the more we can relate with each, learn from each, receive from each. These ideas did not originate with me. But I have experienced them— call it *refined listening*. See what you too can discover on your own exploration of *listening*.

And now you can thank your pets for what they taught you about listening to them.

Chapter 24
JUST LISTEN

I'm not kidding about this title! I know you have heard something titled *Listen* . . . in the last two chapters, and perhaps I mentioned it once or twice in previous chapters :). But there is a point to be made here, and underlined a few times, maybe some brackets, some asterisks, any other highlights you can come up with that gets your attention. This may be one of the most important topics in this book; how well you learn to listen to what is available to you will determine the quality of your life, your connectedness to life, your relationships, your state of health, your state of consciousness, your everything. And I'm still understating the importance of it.

I could just stop here and let you all figure it out, partly because I know you are capable of it, and partly because I would like for you to discover this power on your own with all the hints that have already been provided. Do you recall the wise counsel from my Shaman mentor, Marv, about listening? Would you rather wait for the two by four? There's an easier and quicker way, to getting it, to realizing the value in deep listening, to avoiding the 2 X 4. Spirit doesn't care. It's up to you.

You might notice I'm having fun with this. I wouldn't have it any other way. You can all do this too. There are several keys here to deep listening. We'll review a few.

At first, stillness, calm, quiet, helps, as you tune in. Once you become adept at this you can find yourself in the middle of Grand

Central Station in New York City and find stillness and peace during rush hour. Do you want some of that?

One key is to practice. A lot of us are good talkers, or perhaps more accurately, busy talkers—we talk a lot. It is not a question of quantity of what we say but the quality of what we say and how we say it and knowing how to say the same thing differently to different people. You see we must *listen* to who our listener is. Every listener is different. Every person listens differently. Not many people understand that, perhaps one of the problems in our education system. No one size fits all. Maybe we'll come back to this later. Allow it to marinate for now.

Remember when we discussed cleaning house? We need to empty out the trash, clean out all the junk mail, detoxify, be healthy ourselves, not carrying a lot of our own baggage around to weigh us down or get in the way or to muddy the waters. Then we are not so tethered to stuff and can focus on the things that matter.

This topic is about listening, so it applies to listening here. It applies the same to any other topic too. Become a clean, clear vessel the best you can so you are always at the top of your game, no matter the game, no matter your age—that's just more hidden consensual reality—you decide the game and your age doesn't matter at all, and you play full on no matter what, only as determined by you.

The only other hint I will offer now is for you to discover all the ways you can listen deeply, not limiting yourself to one realm or one world, and then practice, practice, practice. I'd love to be a fly on the wall in your room when you discover this power more eloquently. Since I'm not going to be a fly on your wall, just let me know how this is working for you. If it's as good as I think it will be I will include it in the next book. Do you notice how much of that book is already written with all the contributions I'm anticipating from all you readers?

Now you do not need to listen to me anymore . . . at least not until the next chapter.

Chapter 25
LEARNING TO FLY

Most of us have heard that when a mother bird knows her babies are ready to fly she *assists* them out of the nest, or the curious baby just steps off the edge and finds itself in freefall. If you are a baby eagle you are generally pretty high up. And this is the moment of truth. You either fly or fall. Nature has it designed that most learn to fly when they leave the nest. Will most of you agree?

It is not so different for us human beings. We eventually leave the nest for better or worse, and a whole new world is revealed to us. Most of us learn to fly, and some of us don't.

We have come to a point on our journey together where each of us will be offered the opportunity to fly, higher, further, more skillfully, more artfully on our own, or not. We have explored some of the many tools and powers that are available to us. This is not the last chapter however, so more to come. But it is useful to start anticipating the new world in front of us.

The topics of the following chapters will be interesting and fun for most of us, some maybe challenging, as I will offer some notions of what the unseen world may hold. Some will be dark, or more accurately, address dark things. This is designed to prepare us for our future. Don't worry. There are safety nets, and you are the holder of your own net. Learning how to use your net however is very important. This will be addressed in the following pages.

Recall our conversation on balance, on finding balance, on maintaining balance, or reestablishing balance when we are not in balance. Me too. I am constantly engaged in this balancing act too. With practice we will all get better at this. Now think about our dualistic view of the world. There is up and down, in and out, good and bad, black and white, light and dark, happy and sad, and on and on. Feel free to conjure up as many opposites as you wish, like a game.

Consider there is a non-dualistic approach to life. No opposites, just isness, just things in a state of being, that we are each presented moment by moment, day by day, lifetime by lifetime. There is no in or out, up or down, only you at the center of everything, at the center of your world. There is no black or white, only the existence of color as it shows up to you. This conversation is actually going somewhere so hang in there. And it will have something to do with the world of opposites, and balance, as they exist in our usual domain of awareness.

You see, I believe we inhabit different worlds at different times, and I believe we inhabit more than one world at the same time often. This is just my opinion, and actually my experience too. As usual, you are not required to share it, or buy into it, but do consider it. It may lead you to that higher fruit hanging from the out of reach branches above you. And this is one of the intentions of this book.

By the way, this notion of us existing in more than one world simultaneously is not original with me. I'd like to claim it because it sounds so . . . significant. But it's not. It's just another reality, of which there are many. Since I don't want to lose any of you at this point, just trust this is all leading somewhere. And I know I've presented you with some hard-to-believe stories, and I sense you are now (or have been) veterans of the extreme and unimaginable. And I am pretty certain some of you could share some amazing stories with me too.

Part of learning to fly is the willingness to accept the risk of falling. In the case of baby birds leaving the nest for the first time, the risk of falling can usually mean leaving this world for an experience in another one. Most of us don't know what that looks like yet, but we sense it is different than taking flight in this one and feeling the wind beneath our wings.

170

If we are human, and presumably all who are reading this are human, we have all flown at times—read that as having succeeded or excelled in something—or fallen and crashed. I don't think I need to define either for you with examples. We have all been there, some of us more than a few times. At the risk of a cliché the point of falling is to get back up again. It's a learning experience. Babies do it so well and never complain most of the time. They get back up and keep going. It's life.

But many of us accept a fall as defeat or failure. We stay down, or we choose to not try to get back up again. This chapter could be titled *Learning to Fall* rather than *Learning to Fly*. Has anyone seen this happen to anyone they know? The rest of this chapter will be devoted to learning how to get back up again, and then, learning how to fly in a way only most dream about.

An actual idea I've had for a lot of years was that I wanted to go into senior centers and nursing homes to teach falling. There is a sound reason behind this. As an Orthopaedic surgical resident, I took care of a number of seniors who fell, often fracturing their wrists, elbows, shoulders, or hips, commonly. It occurred to me that if they could be trained to fall properly, they may not sustain the injuries they did. For some they never fully recovered from these injuries, some even dying as a complication of their falls or as a complication from surgery for those injuries.

I've had a lot of experience in falling—from my training in the Martial Arts, from my life as a paratrooper and many parachute landing falls (PLF's) as they are called. All you airborne readers out there know what I am talking about. I've also had a lot of sport parachute jumps (and landings). You can hit pretty hard on some jumps as any jumper can tell you, so it helps to know how to land properly and distribute the forces of that hard landing over your body so one joint or extremity doesn't take it all. High performance canopies make controlled landings safer with hardly any impact, but there is a learning curve to master one.

On one jump into the Florida Everglades on a training exercise with the SAS (British Special Air Service) our group sustained five

171

fractured legs on four soldiers. I helped take care of all of them on the drop zone before rejoining my team for training.

Suffice it to say I've had experience with falling and landing safely. Add that to my bone and joint training in Orthopaedics and I seemed perfectly suited to teach this art to seniors, with their willingness, and proper cushioning, equipment, etc so they would be safe learning. It never happened though. I hope someone reading this picks up on the idea and offers it to a very vulnerable population of seniors at growing risk as they age. And you can continue to teach fitness to them at any age. Just begin. It will be appreciated.

I know I digressed a bit as this conversation on falling unfolded, but that's part of the adventure and spontaneity of creation. Suppose one or more of you took the last few paragraphs seriously and started something for seniors so needed and appreciated. I do know a lot of you are already working with seniors on strengthening and flexibility, a friend of mine for one. Why not take whatever you're doing to the next level then? A whole new niche could manifest. Just imagine the injuries that could be prevented and the joy that could be produced in our senior populations as they gain skill, strength and flexibility in this area.

And I know a number of you are already taking this to the next level, encouraging fitness and movement and suppleness and quicker reaction times to the people you work with on their way to elder status. Inject into this *making this a joyful journey for all with whom you work*, and you are on your way to transforming the lives of others in such a grand way. Just review the mortality and morbidity statistics of all those things that compromise health in our populations around the world and you will quickly note there is much room for healthy changes. Why not be one of those to introduce those changes whether you are in healthcare, or simply one who cares about health?

You can read between the lines of the last paragraph as this is yet another opportunity to learn how to fly. So get comfortable with your new wings and fly, or challenge the wings you already have to fly higher, stronger, more eloquently than they have before.

Now just for the fun of it, make a list of all the things that you personally feel would assist you in learning how to fly better, stronger, more eloquently. Do you have to lessen the load, drop some baggage or extra weight that has been holding you back—read that as anything that may be weighing you down and holding you back physically, mentally, or emotionally, anything you feel shackled to that you wish to be free of.

We all have these things. Me too. I am always looking (and listening) . . . What's next to change, to improve, to heal from, to strengthen, to grow into, to become?

. . . and nowadays I allow myself to be free of limitations. And I always ask myself, am I having fun? Fun and joy are important to include whenever possible. Why? Because I say so for me. I enjoy life more when I'm having fun and feeling joyful.

This too is another choice for you. Do you want more fun and joy and playfulness in your life or not?

I used to say, the sky is the limit. Now I say there are no limits. Only the ones that are self-imposed. I tell my patients this too. So, I'm learning to give up all limitations, to live outside the nine dots, to spread my wings even more, to fly higher and better than I ever have before. And this is available to all of us. Are you interested in living outside the nine dots? Are you interested in living totally out of your own design?

I could say more, but given who I am talking to, I don't think it is necessary. I can sense that by the time we've come this far together on our journey, we've already gotten it. I will assert that all of you have already learned to fly—and those of you who were flying before are now flying higher, and those who haven't felt they could fly now see that they can fly and are flying. How can I state this? Because it's one of my intentions in writing this book. And remember, I'm making this all up. You have the freedom to disagree. You have the freedom to choose. You have a choice to accept your flying abilities or not. And some of you are flight instructors or interested in becoming one.

And really, are there any of you not interested in flying?!

Chapter 26
DREAMING

If you've all been noticing, I may have mentioned dreams and dreaming once or twice in the earlier chapters. In fact, it was even mentioned in the preceding chapter on *Learning to Fly*. In fact, learning to fly and dreaming have a lot in common. They may even be thought of as sisters, just like *Love* and *Forgiveness*.

There is so much written about dreams and dreaming, so many courses on dreams and dreaming, and we all (or at least most of us) dream. So we are talking about something familiar and perhaps we have a good foundation and understanding on dreams. Let's leave all that at the door when you enter this room of dreams we are about to enter. Let's start this with a beginner's mind approach.

Before I start, why don't each of you start? How would you start writing about dreaming? Just note that some of you immediately leaped into some ideas about what to say. Some of you hesitated a moment to consider the task. Some of you may have felt, "Whoa, no, not me. I can't do that." . . . pretty much like the baby eagles stepping out of the nest for the first time, most fly, some don't.

Like the chapter on flying, all of us were challenged to fly, to fly higher, better, etc. My intention is that we all fly. In this chapter it will be about much more than a familiar experience called dreaming. It will be about dreaming for sure, and it will be about designing our dreams as we desire them, and then turning them loose perhaps with the power for them to manifest as we wish.

Star light, star bright
First star I see tonight
I wish I may, I wish I might
Have this wish I wish tonight

How many of you recall this nursery rhyme? Is a dream a wish, a wish a dream?

Dreams, wishes, desires, longings, wants . . . Let's place all these things in one basket and call them, *Things we would like to have, be, experience, etc in our lives,* okay? For simplification—remember, I like simple—we could just call them all DREAMS. So perhaps we come full circle to arrive at simply . . . DREAMS.

Why I took the time and space to say that last paragraph was to simply embed the images that anything you desire, wish for, want, in your life is covered under one word, Dreams (or its action form, Dreaming). You choose. In fact, if you like another word more than dreaming, feel free to make it up. And this is exactly what this chapter will be about, **Dreaming OUR World Into Existence**, perhaps exactly like we dream it and desire it to manifest.

This notion of dreaming our world into existence is also not new to me, as I mentioned it in an earlier chapter when referring to what the Q'ero of the High Andes, are doing, and have been doing for a long time—dreaming their world into existence so their children's children (and our children's children) are born into a better world. You'll have to come back to see if this happens. Or better yet, trust that it is already happening, and you can be part of it.

We are coming to the realm of the Mythic, the world Shamans like to play in, and engage others in on their journeys. Not much can be proven for you scientific-minded types here who need proof for the existence of something. So I will just encourage you all to join in the fun anyway and see what shows up for you.

Many of us have had exposure to dreams, dream interpretations, in addition to our own dreams. Most of us are aware we can dream while asleep or dream while we are awake. Most of us have heard of daydreaming, and in fact probably most of us have daydreamed. If you have ever wished for anything you may call that a daydream also. Has anyone ever been less than enthusiastic about a class in your school and found your mind wandering to another place, time, or activity. Feel free to call this a daydream. I confess, I've been there once or twice :).

Let's explore what it may take for our dreams to come true, for our dreams to manifest, for our dreams to become a reality. I'll take a guess that many of us have had the experience of at least one of our dreams coming true, or if not us personally, we know someone or about someone who has had their dream come true. Does anyone doubt that some dreams do at some time, at least for some of us, come true and manifest? Recall that I said earlier that this book grew out of a dream I had.

Now if any of us know that dreams can come true, then we also know there is possibility for each of us manifesting a dream. I am going to suggest right here and now that we all develop the skill and awareness to harness (and maybe. harvest) our dreams. Suppose we can create a dream at will, and then bring it to life for each of us? Just for the fun of it, assume this is already so now—that you are a Dream maker, soon to become a Dream Master. What constitutes becoming a Dream Master is simply demonstrating that you are creating your dreams—that you are realizing your dreams. Anyone interested in this? I thought so!

This is a good place to introduce the notion of the power of our thoughts and look together at what we think and how we think, and decide if it matters. You will all have to weigh in on those questions and decide for your Selves. I will share my thoughts now.

I have looked at this for a lot of years, have read a lot about it, and have journeyed deeply within and without to arrive at where I am now. I absolutely believe there is great power to how we think, invoke our thoughts, and create our futures based upon those thoughts. Think of thoughts as the seeds of creation. And we as the thinkers, can come up with any thought of any design of any creation, plant them in fertile soil, and watch them manifest. That stated, I will also suggest that many of us squander this ability, this power, in the living of our lives. This is where the term, living mindfully, springs forth (for me anyway).

I will suggest that this process has been in place since the beginning of time. Some of you may have heard that this whole universe manifested itself from the thought of an all-knowing, all-powerful formless cosmic energy that had the desire (the thought) to manifest itself. Most of us have heard of the Big Bang Theory on the creation of the universe . . . Nothingness . . . then a big bang and there it was, the universe in its infancy of manifest creation, and then evolution as we understand it. Hard to wrap my head around, but somehow what we've got now arrived somehow, or was always here. Part of the great mystery. Actually, the beginning doesn't matter anymore. It's here. We're here. And now what?

I've often pointed out to my patients over the years the relationship between matter and energy, represented by Einstein's famous equation $E=mc^2$. Specifically, this states that matter and energy are interconvertible (they can be interchanged). I'll then say that thoughts are a form of energy which we can now measure. So, thinking a thought (energy) about something desired in our physical world (matter) serves to create it, possibly through a chain of specific events. Maybe we can influence what shows up for us. Maybe we help bring it about. So what are you thinking about these days? Choose your thoughts as if they matter (no pun intended) because they do.

I could go on and on about dreams and dreaming but at this point I will turn it all over to each of you. Let me suggest you start practicing right now in dreaming your life into the reality you wish to manifest. And it you are already doing this, then perhaps someone else would appreciate your guidance. One of my dreams is to see the whole world doing this eventually.

What are you dreaming about right now? . . . Yes, hold that thought! That's a dream in the making.

Chapter 27
IMAGINATION

I don't know about you, but Imagination seems to just naturally follow Dreaming. Like it may take imagination to dream something into reality. Like to dream big— my suggestion while we're playing at this—it may take quite an imagination.

We've talked about this before, and I suspect most of you are pretty adept at imagining. I will ask much more of you in this chapter. Don't get nervous about this request . . . It is, after all, your life that I wish to be magical and exceed your wildest dreams, your wildest imaginings at this time. So for now, just get used to this idea. I'll give you until the next paragraph to prepare yourself for this.

Are you ready?! You see how much I ask of you? Remember, we are living in timelessness, at least in this world we are creating together. Time is relative. Just ask Einstein. Don't worry about the fact that he has left his body in this reality. He will still respond to you.

Perhaps some of you will note, imagination is at play here. And it is absolutely so for me too. I like to walk my talk. For the record, I am having a conversation with Einstein right now. He is very pleased this conversation is taking place right now. This just furthers what he was putting into the world with his work. And if you doubt what I just said, recall that I am making this all up. But also consider that I am not.

All that is left for this chapter is for you to recognize what you already possess. For some of you this may take a stretch of your imagination, but that's the whole point of this chapter. Now recognize what is within you, recognize your power, put it to good use, and create the life you have been dreaming about. No limitations! Do you recall me saying that before?

And I fully expect to hear from at least a few of you about what you've dreamed up, and what you've created in your life because of this conversation. By the end of this story, I will have information for you on where to send your thoughts.

Chapter 28
INTUITION

Earlier I promised you a chapter on imagination and one on intuition. It is possible to think of these two as sisters too. They draw upon the same source. They are not part of our tangible physical reality but may assist us greatly in creating our manifest reality at any moment we choose to engage them.

This could be a very short chapter too if you just choose to listen to Marv and accept his assertion about imagination . . . it's like talking to God. I would suggest that the same source applies to intuition. Where does all that good stuff come from otherwise?!

And how good it is, is up to each of us to determine depending upon how we interpret what shows up for us in our lives. If you take my word for it, you can bank on the value of these two qualities. But then you recall that I've told you not to trust a word of what I tell you. So once again, no life raft to cling to. You will have to arrive at your own conclusions. But I will add that I've spent a few minutes of my life on these topics and have noticed they are of enormous value and have proven so in the lives of many over a very long time.

We've discussed the mechanics of intuition in Chapter One if you recall—your gut feeling, the voice of your internal guru or shaman, your Spirit guide, or guardian angel, whatever you wish to call that voice that speaks to each of us at times. Reread it now if you wish. It's important. It is still your decision whether to listen to it or not.

Remember guidance from this source does not need to be followed. Another choice. I follow mine, and it always makes a difference.

Now, take this chapter, and this topic, and run with it. Lots of practice and continuing refinement is suggested. If you do this perhaps you will discover a goldmine within you . . . perhaps :)

Chapter 29
TOUCH

There were a number of contenders for this next chapter. Touch won. And it is an important topic to be viewed from a number of angles. Yes, you guessed it! The good, the bad, and the ugly. And we will explore together this subject of Touch with a small 't' and a large 'T', just like the self and Self (with little 's' and big 'S') and like with Love with a little 'l' and a large 'L'. Do you recall this distinction, viewing a quality or a thing from its ordinary everyday meaning, distinguished from its higher designation, the one that is free of all the baggage and consensual reality? It comes from a higher place, your connection with Source, it's that simple.

Just for a moment before we launch into this topic, give it some thought and imagine where we are going with this conversation. Good practice. I know some of you are flying already, some are clearly excited about your new wings, and some are still using training wheels (training wings) perhaps. It doesn't matter. We are all approaching this work together with our beginner's minds, so we are all on the same page—pun intended :)

When I look at our world, I see much that is beautiful about touch, much that lifts the soul, the Spirit. I also see much touch that is not this. What do you see?

In our dualistic view of the world, there is good touch and bad touch, healthy touch and unhealthy touch, loving touch and harmful touch, and on and on. In a non- dualistic view, there is only touch. It is up to each of us at the very center of our own worlds to choose what touch means for each of us and then bring that into the world to the best of our ability, assuming we are looking to create a better world. I am not willing to assume that is the aim of all of us—to create a better world. Nice idea but hasn't arrived at 100% yet (my opinion). In our work together we are all aiming for 100%. A WIN/WIN for everyone.

And this subject of Touch is, let's say, very *Touchy*, another intended pun. Notice how some of you may have even cringed at the word. I'm just guessing. I don't really know. I do know from talking to a lot of people over a long time, that this topic produces discomfort for some. Can we all acknowledge this is perhaps so to have a fuller understanding and appreciation of this subject?

I won't specify areas in the world where unwanted and inappropriate touch is perpetrated but I will suggest it exists everywhere in the world, another guess, maybe even a high suspicion. I think it exists and affects many lives adversely. If you recall our conversation of unconditional love, I foretold a very different world than the one we live in if all of us lived out of unconditional love. What do you think? I will suggest the same thing is true about Touch, the higher Touch with a large 'T'. Does anyone need this distinction further explained?

If you have ever been someone who has been touched inappropriately, physically abused, assaulted, or molested in any way, touched in any way that you did not want or give permission for, you know what I am talking about. Those are examples of touch with a little 't'. Or if you have been someone who has touched someone else in any unwanted way without permission, you are on the other side of this two-sided coin. What this chapter is going for is simply increased awareness on touching, or more simply again, treating others as you wish to be treated. What this chapter is also going for is to notice what is missing in the world and bring it. Imagine what this world would be like if this happened globally, in every home, community, country of the world.

So this pretty much covers *bad* touch, unwanted touch of any kind. Perhaps good touch needs less explanation. Hopefully we have all experienced this to one degree or another. It can be pleasant, pleasing, health-bringing, and offers many other beneficial attributes. Hugging, handholding, kissing, caressing, lasting embraces, and lovemaking are all examples of healthy physical touch when accompanied by the right intentions and presence. From the point of view of creating good health and a fulfilling vibrant life, I will suggest that it is also very important to us humans—and to many other living non-human beings.

This segues into those who desire to be touched more but it is not available to them. This proves to be its own challenge to some of us. This may call us out to live life more fully, altering who we are, and becoming who we wish to be. To be sure, this probably affects a lot more people than we think.

There are some groups or organizations who engage in hugging as part of their greetings and good-byes at their get-togethers or gatherings. Some may choose the laying on of hands and get a professional massage. These are starts. Becoming an outgoing fun engaging person is not easy for all. Consider this takes practice too. Just consider this if this is what you desire and ignore it if not interested. Just also consider not crossing any boundaries into the realm of unwanted touch. Consider this is another art to explore and develop. Loving touch as a desire is another art to explore and develop. Consider also there has been much research done on healthy touch and it is seen as very beneficial to most and even healing for many.

I mention this last category of touch—the desire to touch—only because I believe it is this strong desire to touch and be touched that leads many quickly into perpetrating the misuse and abuse of unwanted touch. This takes much awareness and sensitivity to live a life that welcomes others into ours but does not intrude into the lives of others in any unwanted ways. This one area if practiced and perfected could alone heal the world, hence it is worthy of mention and attention.

And as an exception to practice, one only must love oneself unconditionally, and then to recognize that each of us are all part of the universal ONE. Nothing is missing, nothing is needed to be complete. Perhaps a more difficult place to arrive at but one that is clearly attainable. We can all do this.

If we feel particularly challenged in this area until we reach the stage of unconditional love, simply ask, make a verbal request of what you want. It may not be granted, may in fact even be viewed as intrusive by some, but has not reached the level of unwanted physical touch, a much greater perceived violation. Do you see the difference?

This brings us to the next category of touch. I asked earlier if anyone has ever had their heart touched by an experience. Being touched emotionally is yet another quality of being touched. When one's heart is touched it generally means that something moved you in a positive way, a warm heartfelt way. Has anyone ever been touched by an Angel?

There is also emotional touch of a wounding or harmful way. Does this need explanation? Perhaps we have all been here too, been wounded, or did the wounding? You see, just by becoming aware of these various qualities of touch assists us in choosing ways of touching with a large 'T', do we all agree? Now all that's left in addition to becoming aware, is becoming aware NOW in the moment in every moment.

Becoming aware in every moment is so important because it keeps us engaged in the practice of this art of touch, of developing loving touch, of growing the ability to engage in loving touch and nurturing loving touch for the rest of our life. This becomes like the 100th Monkey phenomena. It may just spread and infuse the world with this quality we really do desperately need in our world . . . and I do mean *desperately need!*

Once a certain behavior is practiced mindfully over and over again, we become *unconsciously competent* at it—it happens automatically without much thought at all, like tying our shoelaces.

And I am not naïve. I know that most of the people who picked up this book and are still reading are not the ones who generally need to become more aware of *Touch* as we have addressed in this chapter. It is already likely part of your awareness and your behavior patterns. But it obviously isn't for a lot of the rest of the world. So you have your assignment, should you agree to accept it. Or call it your mission. Or call it a fun opportunity to inform and change the world for the better, and you get to pick the way in which you will deliver your message. And do consider the world is in desperate need of gaining this awareness and then practicing it muchly. (grammatical error intentional for emphasis!)

Chapter 30
COMMUNICATION & RELATIONSHIP

Much of the life we share as humans comes down to these two qualities. Many of us are almost constantly engaged in communicating with one another, or relating to one another, and usually both simultaneously. What we will explore in this chapter is not that we all do this, but the quality of our communications that in turn affect the quality of our relationships, and vice versa. And since the intention of our work together is generating a life of extraordinary health and vitality and dream fulfillment, I will suggest that how mindfully we communicate and relate with one another makes a big difference in creating this amazing life. Does anyone disagree with this notion? No worries if you do. Stay tuned.

I know that once again I could present the distinction of little 'c' and big 'C" communications, or little 'r' or big 'R' relationships, but I don't feel I need to anymore. In fact, I will request that each of us this far along in this discussion begin doing this automatically with every word, quality, essence, that comes to mind—that is, let's aim for becoming unconsciously competent at expressing ourselves from our Higher Selves—consider becoming a direct channel from Source. It would be something like engaging one's mind before opening one's mouth, as we've all heard the value of, however I will modify that suggestion that we each open our hearts before opening our mouths. And remember, from the wisdom of Ayurveda, the mind is in the heart.

I suspect we have all had the experience of being well communicated to, and not so well communicated to too. We know when communication works and when it doesn't. Like relationship, and relating, we know when it's going well and when it isn't. Often, we don't make it very important and do little about it. But perhaps it leaves a little hook or a barb in us that we carry with us, that even has the potential to fester. It is for each of us to decide if we wish to be complacent about ordinary non-fulfilling communication and relating or not, or even to endure harm-producing communication or relationships, or not. This is another opportunity for each of us to become the change we wish to see in the world.

Does anyone notice any communications issues in the world of today? Any problems with the ways we are relating to one another? If you feel that there could be an entire book on this subject, I agree. In fact, I'm sure a lot have been written on the subject. What would it look like if one of you readers wrote a book in a way that covered these subjects of communication and relationship in a way that they have never been discussed before, in a way that truly made a difference in the world? Perhaps out of a whole new paradigm of communicating and relating? I sense a challenge in the making. Anyone up to it? The world truly needs a fresh look at this arena.

Many of you may have noticed that I have been applying broad strokes and splashes of color to these topics and leaving much of the canvas for you to finish, your choice of supplying all the fine strokes and nuances of color and texture to how you wish to express your Self. I see each of us as particularly gifted with this creative spark that stems from this fire that burns brightly within, recognized by some, maybe not by others, yet.

There is so much left unsaid on communication and relationship because I wish to leave the rest to be stated by how each of you would like the world to appear and begin designing it, but more accurately, begin living it.

A simple guideline to follow for starters is: *Say what you mean, and mean what you say, always with integrity.*
Meet you in the next chapter . . . but first a poem.

THE SENSE IN RELATIONSHIP

Speak softly and kindly
  As if you are talking to a friend who is dying
  Afterall, we are all dying

Listen to others as if your life depended upon it
  Because it does
   Or at least the quality of it

Meet the eyes of others with an open
 heart and a smile
  Hold the gaze for a moment
   This is seeing yourself in
community

Touch gently, touch lovingly, touch more
 With your hands and your heart
  And allow touch back like this in kind

Smell the fragrance of life and living fully
 It is all around us
  And is simply waiting for us to notice

Taste the many flavors of Life
The many textures, the qualities
Savor them . . . a banquet awaits

When you find yourself deviating from this path
Just take note and return to it
It is the way of healing for our World

And with practice perhaps we will get it right.
• • •

John Mills

Chapter 31
SOME THOUGHTS ON DARKNESS AND DARK THINGS

Perhaps the last chapter led us into this one. It did me, as the subject needs to be discussed for the sake of completeness, lest we all walk around the hippopotamus head lying in the center of the living room floor and no one seems to notice it or comment on it. We tend to avoid mention of things we don't like to look at or acknowledge. This becomes a thing like fear, the more we avoid it the more likely we are to attract that thing we fear most to us—as it is has been stated by more than a few. You can form your own opinions on this.

So, let's confront and embrace this notion of darkness and how present it is in our lives. Most of us probably prefer not to be controlled by our fears, or by things that live in the darkness, and maybe it is important to embrace these things as realities, as if there is something for us to learn.

To be sure terrifying and horrendous things happen in our world with regularity. We often do not know why. I do believe dark forces and things are part of our world. Some of us have personally experienced these things or know people who have. My training in the Medicine Wheel of the Shaman's Altar brought me deeper into this awareness. Sorcery exists—the dark side of Shamanism—and it is the work of some Shamans to work with those afflicted by sorcery. I will not say much detail about it but will say that I believe whatever can be imagined, good or evil, can be. We can choose through a dualistic world view of opposites. All can exist, limited only by our imaginations.

Or we can adopt the notion of non-dual existence. Things are or are not in our experience at the center of each of our worlds. Then we can be according to our choosing, our desires, our dreams. We each decide for our Selves.

In my Shamanic world we each are eventually given protections through a set of rites that keep us safer from dark forces and dark things. It is said that once a Shaman, we become a beacon drawing unwanted attention to us from the dark side. I don't know, but I sense this is so. This reality is not something I fear. I do respect it though. And I willingly cohabit this world with all that is in it, doing my part to the best of my ability, forming alliances and relationships wherever.

As I understand it, the only difference between a Shaman and a Sorcerer is their intention. Their abilities are the same, but one uses his or her powers for good and for healing purposes with pure intent, and the other for selfish purposes for profit and power and personal gain, intending harm to another or others. A powerful Shaman can undo the work of a Sorcerer and bring relief to the one afflicted. I have no further details on this that will be shared at this time.

What I will offer is that we each have personal powers sufficient to usually protect us from harm, but this too takes training and practice and awareness. The simplest path perhaps is to get comfortable with our own powers and watch them grow, learn to dream and design our dreams as to what we wish to manifest. This may sound fluffy, but we've covered enough in the early chapters to give each of us some confidence and encouragement to live life by our own choosing.

As for me personally, I have experienced dark things in my life. From each one I chose to see the gift in it eventually (and not always at first), grow from the experience, and allowed my life to be ever illuminated by the experience. This will be different for each of us, allowing for our individual uniqueness.

As a take home message at this point on darkness and dark things, perhaps our own fears are the greatest darkness. If our own thoughts can manifest anything perhaps begin with purifying these. I don't know. I do know I want to leave you all with something useful on this subject, something you can begin working with. It is possible we are living in a world of darkness now when we look around us, and any light we can bring to it will make a difference.

AT HOME IN THE DARK

Like the illusion of darkness
It is what we don't see
That really matters

Some night, tune in
To all that's around you
To all you think you can't see

Begin the experience by first listening
Then feeling the night
The sensations in your body

Notice ripples, currents, waves
Notice what's beneath that
Now notice what's beneath that

Allow yourself to take flight
Join the winged night creatures
What do you see now?

Become the sound
From nearby rustling leaves
And what do they hear?

Is that water flowing?
From whence and to where
Undeterred by obstacles

Do the trees fear the dark
The grass, the wind, the rain
I think not

And the night animals or the insects
Fearing only for a moment
When caught . . . death too is part of life

Yes, darkness and the night
Have much to teach us
If we only pay attention

John Mills

Chapter 32
NATURE

I think the poem ending the last chapter was a perfect lead in to this one. Nature. Nature is, well, after all, everything. And we are Nature too. Consider we too are everything. We are all connected to everything else. Exciting thought, isn't it? Again, another one you can choose to embrace or not. I do. It works for me. You choose for you.

Consider everything in the universe is connected by say this gigantic spider web, every single part of the web in contact with every other thing in the universe, such that when anything causes movement on this vast web, it causes movement on the other side of the universe by virtue of its web connection on that side of the universe. I have heard this analogy before, so I am just passing it on to you. I like it. On a smaller scale, think how a spider knows when something has been caught in its web . . . it feels motion, movement, and then, it's there, capturing its prey! I've watched this. Fascinating. Can you imagine this on the scale of the universe. Take a moment to do this now.

There is so much to be said about Nature that I won't say much more at this time. I have already said a bit, making frequent references to Nature and our relationship with her. More important is leaving it up to your personal discovery, so rich and diverse is this journey. Words cannot begin to define it. But do take the time to explore this vast treasure we live with and within. What I will do is add some of my poetry at the end of this chapter because it says better how Nature has influenced and affected me by virtue of my deepening relationship with her over the years.

I will also mention that we humans have created huge distractions in our lives to keep us from this treasure. If we look at only our digital existence, we can readily see the distractions we have built up with the growth of technology. Not that technology is not a good thing, but as the wisdom of Ayurveda says about it, all things in moderation. It is my opinion we have gone far beyond what may be best for us. The internet, our cell phones, TV, the media, the overwhelming number of opinions of many that try to influence the course of our lives, intentionally or not, are keeping many of us from experiencing this deeper experience of our Selves and all Nature can teach us.

This will be left up to each of us as to how we discover new paths to health and healing and a relationship with Nature which has never left us. We have left her. She simply stands by patiently waiting for us to notice. There is a reason we hear so much about the importance of reconnecting with Nature. And there are so many ways to do this, an infinite number, really. And they will all escape us if we don't take the time to look up—to look up from our cell phones, our computer screens, even from our lives, even from the path we are walking that no longer calls to us. It takes courage to change. It takes even greater courage to change the world for the better. I'll include a poem about this at the end, among others. It is called *Get off the Couch!*

I talk to Nature all the time. And Nature talks to me. If this sounds strange perhaps you haven't tried it yet or taken the time to listen to her many voices. Whether it is a blade of grass, a tree, a flower, a stream or the ocean, the wind, a sparrow, a bee, or anything that catches our attention, all of life is willing and waiting to have a conversation with us. All of life has something to say to us, perhaps something to teach us. The more time we spend with her, the easier this gets for us.

What is yet to be revealed to you will astound many of you, even as you just begin to dip your toes in. And if you are willing to get wet, to truly immerse yourself in this world . . . well, just let me know what

196

you've discovered. It may appear in the next book. This is worth sharing with the world.

And now I will leave the rest of this discovery up to you . . . other than some poetry Nature shared with me which I will now share with you.

DANCE OF SOULS

Like Butterflies
We Humans flutter
From one life experience
To the next

Landing briefly
Partaking of the nectar
Moving on

Recall the caterpillar
Becomes the butterfly
Who brings another form of beauty

And what next
For this winged creature
When fluttering is done

Maybe we are butterflies too
Always moving on
A dance of souls

I will save the next dance for you

. . .

John Mills

GET OFF THE COUCH

It's time you know
To wake up
To stretch

Mother Earth needs water
And nourishment
. . . and nurturing

She needs more flowers
And new flowers too
. . . be a new flower

And don't forget the rest
The rest called 'everything else'
. . . be that too

There is much to be done
Some work for sure
but more play really

Be a catalyst
Be present
Be anything you want

But most important
It's time . . .
Time to get off the couch!

. . .

John Mills

GOING UNNOTICED

Do you ever notice?
How much you don't notice
How much is missed daily
What didn't you see today?

We see a beautiful sunset
Horizon on fire with red and orange
reaching upward into a Persian sky
Clouds a pallet rich in pastels

We pause to watch a Monarch butterfly
Alight on a flower vibrant with color
Then flutter to the next
And again, sometimes

We may gaze at a meandering stream
A rainbow sheltering the distant tree line
Foaming surf crashing on pink shores or
black rocks
Exclaim the beauty of the moment

But what of the cloudy overcast dreary day
Or the weeds around the flower
Or the mud along the stream
Or the dead crabs washed ashore

This is life happening too
Did we see it?
Were you paying attention?
Did you ever go unnoticed?

And how was that for you?
* * *

John Mills

IN THIS PLACE

I live in slow motion
at times these days
not by intent
but by circumstance

In a place of pain
and uncertainty
I vaguely recall what it was like
when not

I yearn for the return
of health, vitality, strength
knowing it is possible
with the right stuff

So I had to look
do I have the right stuff

Perhaps it is a question
we all consider
when facing dissolution

I look to Nature
for her wisdom
Yes, she tells me
You have all you need

Begin now to rebuild
to grow anew
to refresh
just like I do

John Mills

THE DIVERSITY OF WE

Wind rushes by
lifting me a little as
I help lift
this eagle fly

Green everywhere
high walls veins
a spiderweb of chlorophyll
as I walk upon this leaf

Wet dark soil and stone
no light here yet
but after my tunnel
perhaps a little

Rocks a grotto sand
flashes of color
transparency almost
oh to be sea

A whisper of dampness
puffy gray whiteness and some blue
formless with form
ever changing

Flowing with direction kinda
obstacles unknown
I just go around
Freedom is mine

These things I am
these things we are
take a moment
to experience wonder

Then
tell your story

John Mills

SOMETHING TO DEW

This morning
Do something unusual
Take a bath in a dew drop Notice the radiance
Of the earth and the sun within

. . .

THE SNOWFLAKE

The falling snowflakes
 Landed on my hand
  In silence

No . . . Not in silence
 There was a sound
  when I listened more closely

Today it was snowing again
 Again I watched
  Snowflakes falling

Today one of them
 Had something to say
  I listened closely . . .

She said, "Walk like me
 quietly and softly . . .
  bringing beauty, purity and joy
   wherever you land"
  • • •

THE CROOKED TREE

Some see deformity and ugliness
 And some see artistry and beauty
  in the shape But be aware
   either way the tree doesn't care

• • •

203

LOST

Reaching Searching Striving
No . . . Grasping
for a Life fulfilled

Under which rock or stump
or blade of grass
does it hide

Then again
maybe not there
not at all

then where to look
the sky or amongst the clouds
and the birds

No not there either
maybe in the ocean deep down
unreachable

Years go by
You awaken one day
Ah, there it is!
in my heart

THE JUNGLE

I am in a jungle
of beauty
and emotions

Huge leaves
bowing down
to kiss the stream below Soft
gently dancing in the wind
so very green and alive So vocal

And so unlike the waterfall
cascading beneath
reveling in its own music and rhythm

Such contrast
such tranquility
and wildness

Like my emotions
like my heart breath
on fire and not

Turbulence and tranquility
beheld in a single gaze
I feel it It feels me
This contrast this disharmony
is in perfect harmony

It is like me
it informs my life
it is my life
It is me

My work this time
is to adapt
to allow to understand
to share to be with it all
Maybe just to be

That is enough
that'll do
This already is Heaven on Earth

Isn't it, my Beloved

This is what we are
and so it shall be
always and forever

PASTEL MORNING

An artist struggles
To paint
Just the right amount of light
And the absence of light
And color

The photographer confronts
What time of day (light) and
what angle (shadow)
Aperture setting Shutter speed
Which filter
And color

This morning was done in pastels
This could not quite be captured
On canvas or by lens
Breathtaking

Truly, Nature does it best
And we are privileged to witness
The beauty of her creation

FROM THE SHORES OF KAUA'I

I watched the waves
playing with the coconut on the sand
at my feet

Tumbling it and turning it over and over
back and forth
in and out

and then the ocean claimed it
. . .

My heart has been tossed about
like a piece of driftwood at sea
then I notice nothing happen
to the wood
it just enjoys the ride
. . .

Shhhhhhhh

Do you hear it
what the sand is whispering
to the tiny waves
washing over it

Come into my heart my love
I welcome you
and we are already so close
. . .

208

Each wave is the birth of something here
no two alike
gaining size and power
then washing over the satin beach
and then

disappearance
. . .

If I look with my Spirit eyes
I do not see where ocean meets sky
or where land meets water

I see a landscape of particles
held together by love
I see a canvas
that only God can paint upon

Then God tells me I can paint on it too
What does that mean
. . .

John Mills

Chapter 33
POEMS OF LOVE AND DREAMS

We began Part II with Love. Love is calling for more representation. I believe this is because it is such an important quality for we humans to bring more fully into all our lives. Dreams play a role here too and are also requesting to be included. So they will show up in this chapter as well.

I love talking about Love. And I've discovered that the subject lends itself to poetic expression, hence you will all be presented with some more of my poetry. I will suggest that each of you write about Love too, prose or poetry, your choice. Why? Because I think we are running on a shortage of expressing Love and Dreaming in our world (from the Large 'L' and Large 'D' categories). And I think each of us are up to bringing more Love and more Dreaming into our world. This is completely voluntary.

I will assert that if we each write about Love, share Love in the world in whatever way calls to us, that we will experience more Love for ourselves. And I also feel strongly this will bless us with good health, perhaps even great health, vitality, and contentment, and healing too. We may even have more fun and joy in life too. Anyone want to play in this arena? We need more players here—players in Love and Dreaming. Interested?

I have been blessed with some pretty magical experiences in my life. I believe there can be overlap between Love and Magic. The next chapter will be on Magic, specifically *Magic, Miracles and Alchemy*. Nevertheless, I hope you will perhaps experience the Magic in my poems on Love and experience the Love in my poems on Magic. And feel free to join me at any time and write your own as you read mine . . . if it gets you in the mood. And reread Chapter 13 on Poetic Reflections. *We are all poets if we choose to be.*

WANDERING THROUGH THE STARS

As I walk this way
I look back
  My path has been mostly straight
  And sometimes crooked too

And as I look ahead I wonder
What lies beyond
  that distant bend . . .
    I know not, nor does it matter

What does matter is that now
I am here with you
  and always will be
    as we walk the rest of
      the way together

· · ·

John Mills

OPENING

Shimmering
  The veil parts
    A glimpse

Then Freefall
  Joy in space
    I see you
      Caught

By hands and heart
  Gently
    Risking
      Courage, strength
        Present

Embracing
  So warmly
    The soul of another

      At Last

                              John Mills

WILDHEARTS AWAKENING

Starting each day
with a smile
the image of a reflection
of a reflection

You come to mind
in all the richness
of a finely textured dream
sought for so long

Eyes that behold
one another's in love
eager bodies yet
to be explored

A heart and soul
I know so well
and one who knows mine
like I hers

What of this union
of two beings
creating a relationship deeply
committed to one another

So much has been shared
since our first meeting
And now I walk out of my dream
and into ours

John Mills

FIRST KISS

Before this
Before our first kiss
I want our lips to touch
To get to know each other
Lightly
Gently
Softly feeling each other
Without kissing
No hurry no rush
Just the pleasure of touch
And warmth
Held in our lips
But coming from our hearts
Then
And only then
When the time is right
In that time or another . . .

Our First Kiss

. . .

John Mills

215

STAIRWAY TO THE STARS

This climb we are on
This upward spiral
This ascent

Filled with wonder
Delight
Awe
And maybe fear too
The unknown
The risk

To fall
How far down

But what if
We fall up

What if
We lose each other
In the clouds

But what if
We find each other again
Amongst the stars

John Mills

THRESHOLD OF HEAVEN

In knowing you
You have brought me to the threshold of Heaven
Only to discover that God is within me
And that Heaven has always been where I am

John Mills

. . .

MOONSTONE

It was in a dream
that I found it

It was a silk-smooth stone
that glistened in the light

as I picked it out of the water

it reflected the light from the full moon above
and from its twin in the water

the moon always connects my beloved to me
a scarlet cord stretching from my heart to the moon's
and back down to hers
this I know

can you picture it

I brought the stone to my lips
smooth, satiny, wet
a Moonstone kiss
just like my beloved's

. . .

John Mills

A BEND IN THE RIVER

So this is where we are
Life has brought us to this bend in the river
The Elbow it is called at Riversong
and I am crossing it at the junction of rapids
between the upstream masculine part
joining with the downstream feminine
and I feel it
this joining of the two
within me
and beyond me
and both are me
and both are not me

This place is sacred
my friends at Riversong tell me
and I already know this
I feel this union
with the waters of the river
and the sacred
and what lies beyond
what is to be my life from this day forth
shared with another soul
and with the many souls we touch
this journey we are just beginning
is neverending

I am blessed
we are blessed
what speaks to me
to us
is available to all
if we only listen

John Mills

. . .

NO CHOICE

In this experience called Life
We like to think we have choice
An infinite number in any moment
Not so really

Does the Sun have choice in shining?
In bringing light and life to the Earth
In creating dawn every pre-sunrise
And dusk after every sunset

In warming us on a cloudless summer day
At the beach
Or coaxing new grass out of the ground
In the Spring

Do flowers have choice in blooming?
Or fruit ripening on the vine or branch
Or water flowing downstream
Or tides rising and falling

Such is true about my love for you
I do not choose to love you or not
I simply love you
Choice is not part of it

Can I choose to not love you when I do?
Some may say yes
I say no
It is just the way it is

So when you ask the sun to choose not to shine
Or water not to flow
Or plants not to grow

It goes against Nature and is not possible

Like my love for you

. . .

John Mills

SOULTREE

We have spoken
  You and I
    Of our closeness
      To trees and nature

We have spoken
  You and I
    Of our closeness
      To each other

Together we have looked
  At how much
    We are like the trees
      And are like each other

Our roots go deep
  Over many lifetimes
    Our branches reach out
      And touch Heaven

Side by side
  Our roots comingle
    Our leaves caress one another
      We touch in many ways

Together we stand strong
  Supporting each other
    In sunshine and fair weather
      In stormy tempest and heavy wind

Our shadows
  Cast far and wide
    Falling upon those we love
      And those we intend to

Seeing light amidst our leaves and branches
Feeling our roots go deeper every day
We glimpse what lies beyond
As clarity approaches in every way

And what nourishes us? . . .
Why, it is God and Spirit
For we are children of the Universe
We trees and lovers

. . .

John Mills

WILL-O'-THE WISP

You are like a Will-o'-the Wisp
an elusive flame
dancing in the night
in the woods and o'er the marsh

A fleeting luminosity in the dark
very hard to follow
as you dance in and out
of my life

But I know something
and perhaps you do too
we are the same light
it is inevitable . . .

that we light up the darkness together

John Mills

WHISPERS FROM APART

Separated by miles
and circumstance
my beloved and I
wait

Days turn into weeks
weeks turn into months
months . . . well, they go on

The wind blows
it carries a sound
not the wind
but a sound riding on the wind

I listen closer
It is a whisper
Ah is it your whisper
Is that you?!

Louder please
I can barely hear

"I AM COMING TO YOU!"

Ah that I hear

I wonder
can the wind carry you too to me
Now

John Mills

. . .

DREAMING BIG

If one is to dream
Dream big

If dreams really do come true
Why not be a great dreamer

It has been said
That awake we are still dreaming

It has been said
That we are each a dream within a dream

Maybe we do make it all up
Maybe we should use great imagination

Maybe we should invoke great creativity
If our dreams really may come true

At least sometimes

Maybe we should all . . .

DREAM BIG

. . .

John Mills

JOY

"Joy is the most infallible sign of the presence of God"
Tielhard de Chardin

What is your joy? Or perhaps
What brings you joy? Or perhaps
What has you feel joyful?
Have you ever thought about it?
How does joy show up in your body?
in your mind?
in your heart?
in your life?

I know about joy
I've read a lot about it
I used to think that when I felt good
or happy, that was joy
But it never lasted
I could almost watch it fly away,
evaporate, dissolve
into a cloud and drift out of sight

Sometimes I didn't even have time
to prepare for its departure,
so fast it would suddenly disappear,
like a magic act . . . a cruel magic act

I would think sometimes

This didn't occur to me when I was little,
I don't think.
As I grew not much bigger than very little
I was robbed.
Joy was taken away.

This I do remember.
I didn't call it joy then.

My self just noticed it didn't feel good.
This later was called sad.
It looked like not smiling much
on a little kid's face.
Yes, I remember that

Then I grew up a bit more.
I started to look for happy.
I still didn't call it joy.
I don't think I even knew the word
joy then.

Maybe the first time I recall
using the word was in a song
called Joy to the World.
I still didn't know what it meant.
But I had a sense it had something
to do with happy.

Happy was better than sad.

I preferred the feeling of happy in my body.
As I grew older,
I never stopped searching for happy.
Sometimes I would find it.
I liked it.

But then that old cruel magic act
would come up and poof
it would disappear

That's what my life became about,
feeling happy, feeling sad,
feeling good, feeling bad
Even as a grown-up
Especially as a grown-up

Years passed.

I experienced
happy times and sad times
over and over again.

I still didn't use the word joy much as I recall
My children grew up.

Looking back, I now can say they
brought me a lot of joy.
I didn't call it joy when they were little.
I just loved being with them
and we played and laughed a lot.

I now know that
I was totally caught up
in the spirit of joy
having them in my life as my children.

They were fun.

When did I find joy?
When did I use the word over
and over again?
Well, I know I was reading a lot.

I was still looking for happy that
lasted that didn't go away
Then I met someone
someone with whom
I can say

I felt pure joy in being with
like the joy in being with my children

It was a wonderful feeling in my body.
I felt it in my heart too
We even talked of having
a child and calling her Joya
Her chosen name for our
baby girl yet to be born

Then the joy went away when she did
And then it came back when she did
And then it went away again when she did
This happened a number of times

It was kinda like
joy in joy out
joy in joy out
joy in joy out

Do you get the picture?

It still looked a lot like
not smiling much on a little kid's face
It looked like that cruel magic act again

When joy was in,
the little kid was smiling again
When joy was out,
the little kid wasn't smiling

But I was no longer a little kid
Somewhere somehow
I grew older
I didn't feel older
In many ways I still felt like
a little kid

I saw I had to get smarter at this
get better at it
get good at holding onto joy
when it reappeared I really tried this
It didn't work either.

Somewhere along this path
I heard it was better to find joy
inside yourself
than to seek it outside yourself.

I practiced this.

I had been talking to trees—and getting answers
—for over 30 years
Perhaps I should talk to God
to the Creator of Everything

Ah ha, the magic came back!

This time it was white magic
This magic wasn't cruel
It was good magic.
It was happy magic

I began to sense lasting joy within me
for the first time in my life
no matter what was happening in my life
—good or bad

It was like a door to a dark room
was beginning to crack open
and there was this very bright light
shining in

I opened the door fartherMore light came in
This was a clue
This was a sign
The more light I let in

The more joy I began to feel

It was like the joy I felt
when playing with my children.

It was like the joy I felt
in being with the woman
who I loved deeply and who
I felt loved me deeply

Over time we became even closer
she and I
even more in love
even more joyful

Full of joy
Joyful
Full of Joy
Joyful
Full of Joy
Joyful

And then she went away again
But there was still joy present
A bit different than before
But joy
This woman taught me much and
She led me to my SELF

We are not together anymore
And that is okay

The Gift has been received
Joy is present now
No matter what

Do I dream? I do

I still dream of sharing my life with another
in a loving relationship.
Life with this much shared joy
also needs to be shared with the world.

It is what the world is looking for,
what the world needs
This joy is within me now
It is within my heart

It has gone nowhere except when I share it and then it goes
everywhere

Perhaps I have found God within me
and Spirit is smiling and assures me this is so
I need look no further

"Joy is the most infallible sign of the presence of God"
Tielhard de Chardin

John Mills

. . .

Chapter 34
MAGIC MIRACLES AND ALCHEMY

MA'JISHAN

A person with magical powers
as the dictionary explains it
or
(informal) a person with exceptional skill in a particular area

This would define us
You and I are magicians

And when we combine our magic
our powers are well
much greater
pure synergy
you and I

And what is it we are to do
with all this power
with all this magic gifted us

What are we to create with this Spirit present

Well Everything!
let's create everything
together
you and I
and then give it away

*Do you know what **Everything** looks like?*
I do

Let's be Magicians Extraordinaire together

Perhaps the world is now ready for our magic
John Mills

We are approaching the last few chapters of our book. I chose the term *our* as I truly believe we are on a journey together to some new and undiscovered places. It doesn't really matter that I am the writer, and you are the readers. Let's dispel any notion of separation and go for what we are creating together, a common good and benefit for each one of us and for the good of our world. In fact, the last chapter will be titled *A New World*. We are all part of this evolution, this journey unfolding out of the new paradigm that is emerging. I will share in this last chapter with you some of my discoveries. There really is a lot of new and exciting things happening.

Like the title of this chapter implies, this one will be about each of us creating magic, miracles, and alchemy in our lives. I have been studying all three for some time now, and I have described myself to others at times as a *Wizard-in-Training*. I find this useful so it doesn't scare people away when I describe my Self as this. And it they don't take me seriously, well, that's what most would expect anyway. Some do however—take me seriously. And in fact, I take my Self very seriously. You see, when you say something about your Self, you are then called more into living life as the thing you wish to create, to be, to show up as such. So, I'm a *Wizard-in-Training*. . . really!

Now, none of you have to become magicians, or miracle workers, or alchemists, but I am going to suggest that you consider this, knowing that the magic, miracles, or alchemy that you may create in life, won't necessarily look like anyone else's.

First, dare to be different and dream big. We've already covered the powers of imagination, intuition, dreaming, and the power of thoughts that can create things in your life. We may need some more practice in this area, but some of us don't, and you know if you are already one of those doing this. And remember, pay no attention to consensual reality and the dream breakers in your life.

Some of you have heard the expression *believing is seeing*. More of us are more familiar with *seeing is believing*. I used this expression in a health and wellbeing talk in 1985, that believing is seeing—as when you believe something (a thought) you will maybe later see this belief (this thought) manifest. *You will see it.* I still believe this. I have in fact done this more than a few times. This book is one of them. There are many others in my life. I'm still working on some pretty amazing ones. And I am not the only one who is doing this.

Even though this chapter heading may sound somewhat fanciful, I am quite serious about it :). If none of those notions appeal to you, that's fine. Just move on. But first answer this question. If magic, miracles, or alchemy were real, if they really existed, would that excite you? You see, as we are moving into the creation of a new world, I am asking us all to consider the importance of our imaginations. If you can imagine yourself a magician, a miracle worker, a wizard, an alchemist, I think that's the first step and helps for the task ahead of us, to transform our world and make it a better place for all of us, and I feel this transformation begins within each of us.

I suspect it may be difficult for some of us to have a serious conversation about this topic. Remember this is not only a work of Art in our lives but a work of Fiction. We're making this all up and we might as well have fun with it while we're in this creative playful mode. In other words, it may be easier to pretend being a magician or a wizard at first to get us in the arena—on the playing field—and then become the real thing as we discover how to manifest our powers and be a magician or a wizard.

While we're in this mode of creativity and consideration of magic, let's examine one definition of Alchemy. You may recall, it was once a goal of the alchemist to create precious metals like gold out of lesser base metals. This may still be one goal of the alchemist. The definition I align with is: *Alchemy: a seemingly magical process of transformation, creation, or combination; finding the person who's right for you requires very subtle alchemy.* Read up on Alchemy and pick a definition that works for you if this calls to you. I am now much more drawn to magical things whereas once upon a time I wasn't nearly so aware of this. My life has changed because of this belief. I am always looking into the possibility of bringing magic to life, of creating miracles, and in performing alchemy when the opportunity presents itself.

Consider what your life would look like if you were a magician or a wizard, or one who could create miracles, or someone gifted in alchemy. Next, find something to practice on.

And now for some hints before we complete this chapter . . . two more poems.

MIRACLE CHEF

I'm making a Miracle
and it's certain to be
cause I'm planning it with Creator

It has all the ingredients
that Creator wants in this recipe
wants to see more of on Earth

Racial, religious and ethnic tolerance for all
for all children and grownups
everywhere
love, joy, peace and harmony too
we all need more harmony
well, we all need more love, joy, and peace too

Oh and a deep concern for
and support of Mother Earth
and all her beings

What does it take to create a miracle?
imagination, belief, faith, trust and unconditional love
for ourselves and for all others
you cannot leave out the love

and joy, peace and harmony are helpful too
whether creating miracles
or not.

What else does it take . . .
just you
and an open heart
and a willingness to be in life's kitchen where miracles are made

What miracle do you want to make?
Why not begin one now?

And I'll share mine with you when it's done

. . .

John Mills

MOONSHADOW

This once golden moon Mamakilla
now cloaked in dark blue velvet
and holding Mother Earth's Shadow
so closely

Looked quietly down upon
you and me
as we together
looked back at her

beholding moon and stars
so splendid
touching us
on this magical night

We two heaven gazers
so close together apart
beheld each other too
in this moment of no time

Our party of two both agreed
what a magical life
perhaps we are becoming
magicians

And the stars
and the moon
and the shadow
agreed

John Mills

The Magicians
Kim & John
Lunar Eclipse

Chapter 35
A NEW WORLD

Have most of you been holding your breath?! This chapter is your blank canvas. It is your opportunity to design, construct, create the exact world you would love living in, and the one you would love to see your loved ones living in, and the one you would love to see your children's children living in. Just writing those words gets my juices flowing! What do they do for you?

This is where the rubber meets the road. This is where we get to notice whether we are gaining traction in our Dreaming or not. This is where we get to put the quality of our life at stake. So it's important.

I know I am going out on a limb here. I'm not sure anyone else is interested in this subject. It appears to be such an enormous undertaking. Is it even possible? I don't know. I do know that when I look around at the world, there is much that needs attention. There is much that needs fixin'. Really, I believe transformation to a whole new world is needed. I think we are in trouble and getting worse—the so- called slippery slope we are on. It'll go quick unless we reverse the direction we are taking. Actually, we need a whole new road map. Actually, we need a whole new way of being with each other. We in fact need a New World.

It doesn't need to take a lot at first, just baby steps. If everyone began to make a small difference in little ways, it could lead to much bigger changes later. I think we humans could treat each other better in lots of ways. Whatever each of us are already doing to make the world a better place—safer, healthier, kinder, more compassionate, more friendly—just do a little bit more. I think this will eventually catch attention, and perhaps catch on. Slowly but surely one of us can become that 100th monkey that tips the scale and spreads to the whole world.

I think the best place to start is with our Selves. We have the most control in this area. If we simply become kinder, healthier, more compassionate, more sharing of ourselves, and love ourselves unconditionally, it could create miracles (my opinion). It takes much more than inhabiting the body of something that looks like a human being but doesn't act human. Does this resonate with anyone?

What qualities would you identify as being human? What qualities would you like to see more of in the world? How would you like to see humans treating each other? This is worthy of consideration?

The part that makes this notion of a new world so seemingly difficult is that this is new territory for most of us, perhaps all of us. What exactly does *A New World* look like? It may be like what a blank canvas on an easel appears to the painter/artist before he adds that first brush stroke. It was something like when I sat in front of an empty first page and decided that I wanted to write a book that would make a difference to many in the world, but how to begin?! It is what any big endeavor of any kind appears to anyone before beginning that endeavor with no evidence that he or she will be successful at it. This includes a lot of human beings. And we all are aware that many have risen to the occasion and created, well, . . . miracles. But we don't know this until we take the first steps on our path to a Dream and then need to wait until that Dream is realized.

Before we go further together on this business of changing our lives, our experiences, our world, and engage our Selves in creating miracles, what do we do when we notice this isn't happening for us? What if we do not see life showing up (manifesting) like we hope, wish for, dream of? What then? What do we do next?

Curiously, I have experienced this in the past, and am experiencing it now. It is why I am addressing this as we look together at the creation of a new world and what that may take. We need only look at those who have been successful in the past, the trailblazers who came before us, the ones we now can see created miracles themselves in this arena called Life. There are many. There are many stories. Pick one or more that give you hope, encouragement, coax you on to continue whatever endeavor you are about. What I have personally learned is the importance of persistence, of not giving up. And if our goal is a worthy one, I feel we get help, lots of help, from that unseen world we live in. And yes, this brings up the importance of trust, and trusting whatever comes up in our lives.

If we believe that things may not be happening on our personal timeline--our needs, wishes, desires, of the moment—and consider that some greater good awaits us by this delay, then we only need patience and to maintain our intention and vision for what we wish to create. And for me it also required faith and trust. I also notice that when it is happening to me—like now, and one reason I am writing about it—that patience and trust always pay off. Whatever was happening emerged from the shadows, became clearer with time, and manifested as a thing of value and joyful discovery later. It's also just more of looking for the silver lining to the dark cloud, knowing that the sun is always shining somewhere, and I trust that it will shine on me again.

This may not be a formula for success for you, but I notice that the more I apply it to my life, it works. This is just more for each of us to consider and to experiment with in this grand laboratory of life.

This notion to trust that our desires will be eventually fulfilled no matter what isn't new. I am not the first to come up with this notion. Others have stated it. As Deepak Chopra puts it in his book *The Seven Spiritual Laws of Success*, everyone's desires will be fulfilled by Spirit *when the season is right.* I read that as it is Spirit's decision when the timing is right to grant our wishes, desires, and dreams, not based upon our whim in the moment. Maybe Spirit is looking for commitment, dedication to our dreams, and persistence, before saying Yes. Maybe this is what it means when we speak of *co-creating with God*—the co piece means there is more than me involved in the thing being created.

That something else unseen may be behind our experience of life is something each of us may want to explore and decide upon—and determine how we wish to implement in our life in the pursuit of our dreams, or not. No one needs to believe in a higher power, or Spirit, or God, or whatever name we come up with for the Creator or Source. A belief in nothing is fine. I have heard people teach that there is no value in Hope. If this is true for you, I'm okay with that.

Whether we do or do not believe in Hope, Spirit, or God, or anything really, is up to each of us to figure out. I only ask people with any experience they share with me in a therapeutic setting is, "and how is that working for you?" This gives them the opportunity to look deeper at their lives, since they have come to me for help. I'm not attached to what they come up with. I'm not attached to any beliefs I arrive at either. In my case I stay open to all possibilities and deeper exploration always. I may not agree with someone's particular belief(s) but I will not impose mine on them unless my opinion is requested. *To each his own.*

Some of us believe in God, some of us don't. Some of us believe in angels, elves, pixies, fairies, and other beings most of us don't see. Some of us don't. This is a personal decision, yet we can be surprised at times how strongly someone imposes their opinion on others about *how life really is!* This is what each of us will confront as we work toward a New World. There will be those we encounter who do not want a new world. You see, better or new for some does not exist, and change is a scary thought. This is life. Carry on with your own dreams regardless of the views of others attempting to discourage you. Ask any of those who came before this moment and realized their dreams, even when not popular.

If you just look at all the names of people that I quoted in the chapter on Forgiveness, each has made substantial change in making the world a better place. Each has lived a dream and helped to manifest that dream. If you need a reminder, just reread the chapter. This is what each of us are doing, or more specifically, being challenged to create, as we consider what A New World will look like. And since there is power in **Synergy**, I suggest we could all work together on the creation of a New World, a world that works for everyone, that will be working even better for our children's children, and for Mother Nature herself, if we stay the course.

Synergy is a powerful quality. It is a quality I would suggest we all consider and embrace as we take on together the creation of A New World—a new, healthier, happier, more vital and joyful world, just like I'm suggesting for each of us in our own personal lives. *We are a microcosm of the macrocosm.* I've said that before in my flier on Flying Warrior Training (2014), included below.

And here are some quotes on Synergy from Stephen Covey, an internationally acclaimed writer and speaker. Stephen says:

ON SYNERGY

"When the spirit of synergy starts to come into the relationship you are both looking in the same direction and searching for a third alternative whereby you not only tolerate and accept differences, but actually celebrate them. You value the differing perceptions, feelings, and experiences immensely, for they enable you to create something far better. Creating a third alternative that is felt by each person to be superior to those originally proposed becomes one of the most bonding experiences in relationships and in life."

"If we want to change a situation, we first have to change ourselves. And to change ourselves effectively, we first have to change our perceptions."

"We must look at the lens through which we see the world, as well as at the world we see, and understand that the lens itself shapes how we interpret the world."

"Paradigms are powerful, because they create the lens through which we see the world. The power of a paradigm shift is the essential power of quantum change, whether that shift is an instantaneous or a slow and deliberate process."

"Dependence is the paradigm of you—you take care of me. Independence is the paradigm of I—I can do it, I am responsible. Interdependence is the paradigm of we—we can do it; we can

cooperate, we can combine our talents and abilities and create something greater together. Dependent people need others to get what they want. Independent people can get what they want through their own effort. Interdependent people combine their own efforts with the efforts of others to achieve their greatest success. Only independent people can become interdependent."

"Synergy is everywhere in nature. If you plant two plants close together, the roots commingle and improve the quality of the soil so that both plants will grow better than if they were separated. If you put two pieces of wood together, they will hold much more than the total weight held by each separately. The whole is greater than the sum of its parts. One plus one equals three or more."

"The essence of synergy is to value differences—to respect them, to build on strengths, to compensate for weaknesses."

ALBERT EINSTEIN OBSERVED, *"The significant problems we face cannot be solved at the same level of thinking we were at when we created them."*

. . .

This presents itself as a good time to talk about the works of others who are introducing new ideas and concepts in the construction of a new way of looking at the world, and at the actual creation of a new world. I will suggest that there are many writers, authors, teachers, scientists, researchers, healers, artists—you can name more groups— who have been on this path for a long time and introducing us to the possibilities of enriching our own lives, of healing comprehensively, of contributing to a new and healthier world for all of us.

I will mention in the Appendices of this book, one section titled *Books to Grow By* that I made up as a handout for my patients who expressed an interest in going deeper. In mentioning some of the authors of these works, I fail to include so many more that have been of enormous value in my life—that is, I cannot do justice to all the people I would wish to include among those out there that have made enormous difference in the lives of others and in making the world a better place.

And I know some of you are among this group, and probably all of you will eventually be in this group. You readers are the *movers and shakers,* as the expression goes. You are on the playing field—you are in the game and not spectators on the bleachers, as I mentioned before in a previous chapter. And I did say we are all in this together. I feel I am in good company.

The thread that connects all things to our optimal journey to whatever we wish to create, varies for each one of us. It can be daunting, even overwhelming at times, when we consider the infinite number of choices we have. I have always seen myself as being on a journey of some kind and explored a lot over the course of my life, driven by a desire to experience and learn. As the years passed, this desire never left me, and I began to share what I learned.

What I also began to do was to just trust whatever showed up in my life as exactly what I was to do next. There were clearly some downsides to this, but I began to see the adventure in embracing the unknown. Believe me when I say there were some difficult times along this path. The important thing for me was I began to accept them and believed they too were designed for me. They taught me much and allowed me to grow into who I am. And I eventually got to see that if I waited, I'd discover the reason for the loss, or disappointment, or sadness, and I would always recognize later what the silver lining to the dark cloud was about.

I gained more confidence—the more I experienced the more I trusted whatever showed up as just the perfect thing I needed in my life. Pretty much, disappointments disappeared. It's not like I didn't desire it to be another way at times, because I did. But I became good at asking Spirit why this happened, and I would get an almost immediate answer that was satisfying, that made sense in the grand scheme of my life.

You can see in the preceding paragraphs this could show up as a pep talk . . . because it is! If we are tackling the creation of a New World, it is very important to realize there may be setbacks, breakdowns, obstacles, upsets, disappointment, others who don't agree and resist our vision, rule makers who will say we are breaking the rules, and on and on and on. This has always been so. What we are up to will take courage, strength, fortitude, optimism, synergy, passion, trust, faith, hope, and much patience. Love wouldn't hurt either. You can come up with more descriptive terms if you'd like. There are many more. But you get the idea.

Also consider this may be a lot of fun, to work magic, to create miracles, to be involved with others like us who wish to do this work too, and that perhaps Spirit will support us in unseen ways. Truly a Bilbo Baggins Adventure.

While there are people and organizations around the world doing work of this nature right now, and many who have been for a long time, I will mention only a few out of the great number that exist just to provide examples for the depth and breadth of their creativity. Each was a contribution to me personally.

The Time of the Sixth Sun was offered online a couple years ago. I watched it. There was an introductory movie to it followed by a series featuring several of the guest speakers. The Sixth Sun refers to this new era we are entering—the Sixth epoch or 6th 5000-year time period of life here on Earth. We are entering a new one now, a new era, and a New World experience will be emerging. This one will be created by the *Warriors of the Rainbow*—the Brown, the Red, the Yellow, the White from all over the world coming to work together toward a common goal, toward a shared world, toward the creation of a New World.

Sprinkled into this series was more than a little mention of the role of Shamans from all over the Earth. Shamans are also referred to as Earth Keepers. To be a Shaman, one assumes Stewardship of Mother Earth for all future generations. Many humans are not taking care of Mother Earth. Many do not even care about taking care of the Earth. They only need to learn and understand the importance of taking care of Mother Earth as if taking care of themselves. Unfortunately, many do not take care of themselves very well either. There is still much to be done, much to be learned, much to be taught, if we are going to make it into this next epoch called The Time of the Sixth Sun. One such way is to live by example what we wish to see. Since we are on the topic let's mention a few more things about Shamans. Remember the *Qualities of a Shaman* that were outlined in an earlier chapter. These qualities if practiced are sufficient to create major change in the world if we can all get behind them—that is to say, practice them daily. While Shamanism may not have a corner on the market to create major changes within us and within our world, it is certainly one of the main ones. If any of you decide to walk the path of a Shaman, I'd like to invite you to contribute to my next book to describe your experience.

Alberto Villoldo, PhD is a Medical Anthropologist and a Shaman. He founded the *Four Winds Society* to teach it. He has written a number of books, most of which I have read. *Healer, Shaman, Sage* is among his earlier ones and *One Spirit Medicine* and *Grow A New Body* are the latest ones that I've read. None will disappoint and all will contribute to your understanding of the path. I have talked about the principles of how our bodies replace and replenish themselves with healthy cells and body parts when we are healthy, and not as well when we are a storehouse of toxins and unhealthy cells and organs (and thoughts and deeds). *Grow A New Body* addresses this.

Another revelation Dr Villoldo offers is that we are changing. Humans are in a process of transcending from homo-sapiens to homo-luminous—less physical and more light-bodied. This is an interesting thought. Some of us have heard of light beings. Some of us have heard of these other-dimensional beings that walk among us. Stay tuned to this notion. This could be what's ahead. A bunch of other people have talked of this before. It is for each of us to explore as we desire, and it will help to keep an open mind with a lot of curiosity.

Marv Harwood, my Shaman teacher, who also trained with Dr Villoldo and stays in communication with him, is also writing a book jointly with one of the Q'ero Shamans who we trained with in Peru. Wilbert is a professor in one of the universities in Cuzco. Their book is to detail their work in Shamanism and to write about the merging of the North and the South traditions, that of the Native Americans and the Q'ero— *"When Eagle and Condor will fly wingtip to wingtip."*

Eagle and Condor also represent the masculine and feminine principles in the world—*always the importance of balance being revealed.*

My other Shaman teacher and mentor from my Kimmapii community in Canada, is Shanon Harwood, Marv's wife, and she has also been guiding my Shaman training since I began it. Both Marv and Shanon are elders in the First Nations Blackfoot Tribe. Both were trained by Joe and Josephine Crowshoe, Spiritual Elders of the Blackfoot Nation. They were affectionately called *the Old Man and the Old Woman.*

Joe and Josephine have crossed over several years ago, and Marv and Shanon continue the work of bridging the gap between people—they have been doing so for many years. If you wish solid training as a Shaman, I would suggest doing it with these two.

Shanon has recently written her own book, titled *Currency*. This book is a work of fiction in that it portrays the story of people undergoing a redesign of the way the world works. It is extremely creative. I will not say more about it now, other than to suggest it be read. I mention it because this is what it is going to take for all of us to view the world in a new paradigm. Currency was born outside of the nine dots, but it is a possible world we could create together. Shanon also appears in Part III, *Voices of the Goddess.*

I will now step from the world of the Shaman into the ancient tradition of Ayurveda and speak of Dr Kulreet Chaudhary. Dr Kulreet was born in India and moved to the US at age 4. She trained as a Neurologist in San Diego. and served as the Director of the Wellspring Clinic at Scripps Memorial Hospital in La Jolla, CA for 10 years before moving back to India with her husband and son to Tamil Nadu, outside of Vellore, at the request of Amma, her spiritual teacher and guru.

Dr Kulreet is part of the New World design. I've just read her second and last book, *Sound Medicine*. In it Dr Kulreet noted her neurology patients were not improving under the usual western pharmaceutical regimens for neurological disorders. She noted that

250

this was true for most of her patients. They only worsened with time—my observation also with chronic neurological conditions.

What Dr Kulreet began doing was introducing Ayurvedic wisdom into her patient's care and practice. This included diet and lifestyle principles that I mentioned earlier in this book. Meditation and Yoga were part of her program, and she also introduced her patients to Mantra meditation—chanting a mantra 20-30 minutes twice a day as her patients adjusted to this new approach. Her patients began improving! The sounds and vibrations are deeply healing.

I will not tell her story, so you'll have to read *Sound Medicine* if you want to get the rest of it. I will also tell you from my experience as an Ayurvedic Practitioner, you will discover a gold mine in her words and her work. Visiting Dr Kulreet and her Ayurvedic and Siddha medicine clinic in India is now on my to-do list. Catch one of her pod casts to get a more in depth feeling for her personally. I will simply state that her suggestions for improving the quality of our lives and our longevity will amaze and enrich.

I would be amiss to not mention the *Flying Warrior Training* program created by me in 2014. This grew out of a homework assignment during my training in Ayurveda at Kripalu. We were each tasked to design a flier on what we would each like to bring into the world that would express our Ayurvedic training and what we would offer. This was to be completed by our final class still weeks away. Each newly created flier by all students was to be hung on the walls of our course room for all to see (written descriptions to be attached as desired). This was my blank canvas and an opportunity to dream out loud with my classmates and our teachers. I loved tackling the assignment and I did not skimp on imagination or variety. The flier and written descriptions appear below:

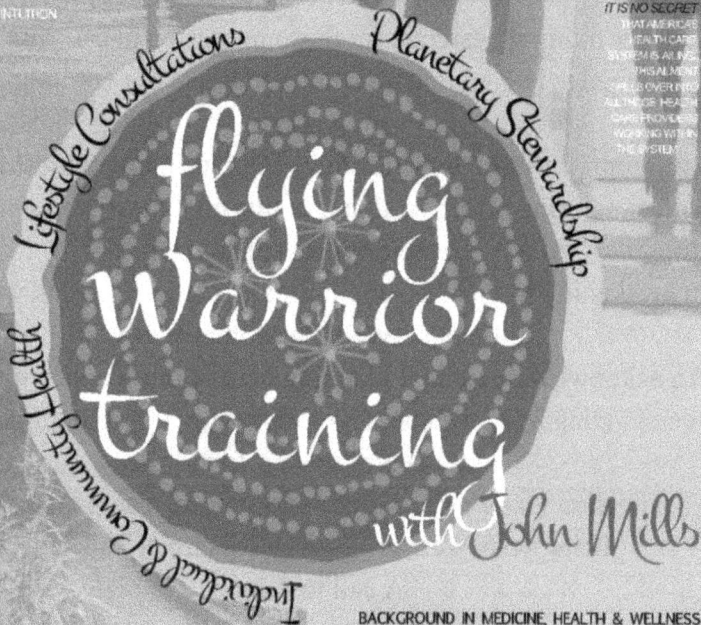

YOGA & AYURVEDA
AN INTEGRATIVE APPROACH

UNDERSTANDING THE IMPORTANCE OF ...
DIET AND LIFESTYLE

WHAT WE EAT, WHEN WE EAT, HOW WE EAT

ENERGY MEDICINE AND QUANTUM THEORY

MINDFUL LIVING

CREATING A LIFE OF PURPOSE ... AND LOVING IT!

ASANA, PRANAYAMA, & MEDITATION
STRESS MANAGEMENT

THE VALUE OF MOVEMENT, PLAY AND SPIRIT

DEEPENING INTUITION

VIBRANT HEALTH
FOR HEALTH CARE PROFESSIONALS

LET'S DISCUSS
WHAT IT MAY TAKE TO INFUSE NEW LIFE, VITALITY, ENTHUSIASM AND JOY INTO OUR LIVES WHILE IN THE SERVICE OF OTHERS

LET'S EXAMINE
WHAT IS NOT WORKING IN HEALTH CARE — AND IN OUR LIVES

TRANSFORMATION IS POSSIBLE ...
ALL IT TAKES IS WILL, COMMUNITY, & EFFECTIVE ACTION

IT IS NO SECRET
THAT AMERICA'S
HEALTH CARE
SYSTEM IS AILING
... THIS AILMENT
SPILLS OVER INTO
ALL OF US - HEALTH
CARE PROVIDERS
WORKING WITHIN
THE SYSTEM

Lifestyle Consultations

Planetary Stewardship

Community Health

Individual & Community Stewardship

flying Warrior training with John Mills

NATURE & YOU
SUCCESS AND SURVIVAL

DEEPENING OUR UNDERSTANDING OF

OUR RELATIONSHIP WITH NATURE

OUR AWARENESS OF NATURE

NATURE'S AWARENESS OF US

AND DISCOVERING A PARTNERSHIP FOR LIFE

BACKGROUND IN MEDICINE, HEALTH & WELLNESS

PROFESSIONAL
Chiropractic Physician
Emergency Medicine Physician
Holistic Health Practitioner
Sports Medicine

COMMUNITY
Medical Director

CERTIFICATIONS
Yoga Teacher
Ayurvedic Family Consultant

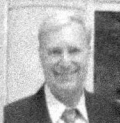

Kripalu

COMMITTED TO GENERATING A HEALTH-FILLED, BALANCED MIND-BODY SPIRIT APPROACH TO LIFE FOR ALL HEALTH-CONSCIOUS HUMAN BEINGS.

RETIRED COLONEL FROM THE US ARMY SPECIAL FORCES, JOHN UNDERSTANDS AND EMBODIES THE WARRIOR SPIRIT — A QUALITY BEING CALLED FOR IN TODAY'S WORLD IF WE ARE TO SURVIVE & THRIVE AS A PEOPLE ... AS HUMAN BEINGS ON PLANET EARTH.

FLYING WARRIOR TRAINING

A teacher training designed for those interested in carrying the torch
of knowledge and enlightenment to others in our communities, our
world
A program for those who desire to embrace the stewardship of our
planet and bring effective action to this goal in whatever way their
creative spirit calls to them
An awakening to the deep and intimate relationship that we human
beings have with Mother Earth
An acknowledgment that in taking care of our planet with a deep
understanding and awareness—of nurturing it—we in turn take care
of ourselves in a profound way
A realization that we are a microcosm of the macrocosm Be Bold!
Bring your Warrior Spirit to the circle. This is . . .
A call to Action
. . .
John Mills

FLYING WARRIOR QUALITIES

Flying Warrior—an asana, a pose in Yoga. What follows here however is far more than a yoga pose . . . it is an exploration of the art of life, of living life artfully, mindfully. Just like we may explore an edge in holding a yoga pose, practitioners know this edge can bring us into a deeper connection with ourselves— with our bodies, with our minds, and in time, with practice, a deeper connection with our spirits, our souls, our atman. As we attune to our bodies, minds and spirits, as we bring them into alignment, we begin to experience transformation. And transformation only happens for the good.

*Of all the poses to choose from in Yoga, why **Flying Warrior**? . . . Because of the metaphor, because of the image within the image—the not-so-hidden deeper meaning. **Flying** can have many associations . . . taking off, soaring, effortless gliding flight on the currents of the wind, seeing from above, a greater perspective of the whole from a height—qualities only birds or people in planes possess by our usual understanding. Yet each one of us can learn how to fly . . . and so we shall.*

__Warrior__ draws one's attention to courage, strength, commitment, protection, discipline, fearlessness, surrender to a higher cause, and supporting that cause no matter what. Our world is in need of more warriors—not warriors on the battlefield where guns and ordnance are used to kill each other, but warriors of the spirit, warriors who know what is Right and can fearlessly take action to do what is Right for the good of everyone, and for the good of our beautiful and wondrous planet.

We all need to rekindle the concept of warriorship (the modern version), the notion that each one of us has unique qualities that can be courageously brought to the forefront of life for the good of all life. Then we begin to breathe life into that awareness, moving us to action, to the actions of a warrior. The time has come. That time is NOW. We possess nothing else in life than NOW, than living in the moment. As Eckhart Tolle has stated, "the past is over and lives only in memory, the future hasn't happened yet and therefore lives only in imagination. All we have is NOW." This is precisely where life is happening. This is precisely where we need to be to begin the rest of the journey.

· · ·

John Mills

We are at the end of this particular journey. Really, it is just the beginning of our journey . . . new map, new compass, new terrain, and perhaps we are new—or at least renewed—in our quests in life, maybe our dreams too. I would venture to guess that we are flying higher now than before. And we are perhaps flying together now—in a formation as an aviator may say—grouped together with a common purpose. I'm excited about our flight plan and who will be in the sky with me. And on the Earth too.

The truth is, I am very excited about the future and all the possibilities before us since we've joined hearts and minds and hands for what lies before us. I truly feel I am in great company and honored that you all stayed with me to the last chapter. So, this is not *goodbye* but just so-long for now. We will continue this journey in the next book for those interested, and for whatever new ventures we may otherwise wish to take on together. I am open to suggestions. And don't forget about dreaming big. Blessings to you all from my heart to yours and may Spirit always be with you and support your every dream.

And thank you all for being a big part of one of my dreams.

THE END
For now

John Mills

PART III
VOICES OF THE GODDESS

VOICES OF THE GODDESS

Introduction To Part III

The idea, the notion, that a Part III was to be, also came during a dream . . . or in that awakening state from a dream. This happened while I was attending another Shaman's Altar training in Canada, this time as a graduate, last November of 2022. I was still in the process of completing this book, still on Part II when this guidance came to add a Part III with the title of Voices of the Goddess offered to me. Hence, Part III was born.

I should state that when things like this occur in my life, I don't question them anymore. I just bring intention to manifesting what has been offered, the Source all you readers of this book are well aware of by now. Of course, I gave deeper thought to why this should be Part III, and that answer presented itself to me immediately too.

You see, we all know we each are half feminine and half masculine by virtue of having in common a father and a mother contributing to our manifestation at birth—you know the XX or XY determinants of our DNA as we once learned about years ago, knowing there are variations on this theme also. For the sake of simplicity, can we just accept this as so? . . . many of us fall into this categorization. If we possess an XX configuration, we are considered female, and if we possess an XY configuration we are considered male. The percentage of each of us that are manifested as more feminine or more masculine in nature is up for discussion on a uniquely individual basis. Can we all agree on this too?

And please recall, no one must agree on any of this, as originally stated in this book in more than one place, remember? For the sake of a conversation about Gods and Goddesses, we are only considering here what is commonly referred to as the feminine, knowing each of us has a composition of both from the point of view stated above. Let's proceed then.

There are also qualities associated with our femaleness and our maleness. Some common feminine traits (which I searched for but also knew off-hand) are Intuition, Empathy, Sensitivity, Collaboration, Vulnerability, Nurturing, Self-awareness, Kindness. There are more. Add as many as you like and which call to you.

For men it used to be "stoicism, competitiveness, dominance, and aggression." These traits are now considered harmful and not accurate. With further research it became clear that we don't know. So many qualities and skills were offered up, none of which got the job done. We are confused about what traits belong to the masculine and seem clearer about the traits attributed to the feminine. Maybe that's part of the problem with the world—largely considered to be run by men, and patriarchal in nature—if we don't know who we are or what we represent.

Two descriptions that I somewhat liked were from Shakespeare and from Richard Phillips. In Shakespeare's *Julius Caesar*, he says about Caesar . . . "His life was gentle, and the elements So mixed in him that Nature might stand up And say to all the world, 'This was a man.'" And one by Richard Phillips in his book *The Masculine Mandate* . . . "Our calling in life really is this simple (although not therefore easy). We are to devote ourselves to working/building and keeping/protecting everything placed into our charge." For me this description fits women too. Women are capable of all this.

It seems women know who they are and mostly show up in the world in their way. Similarly, this does not seem to be so for men. In 2019 President Barack Obama said that the world would be improved "if every nation on earth was run by women (attributed to BBC in a speech he gave in Singapore that year). I agree. I would like to see women running the world.

Perhaps the qualities of kindness and caring and capacity to nurture now attributed to the feminine would be more prevalent and would win over the world's people. Mother Earth would perhaps flourish and thrive. *Curious she is a Mother too.*

And if you need more evidence, just look at the mess we are in in our current world of today, largely ruled by men . . . a simplistic statement perhaps but not necessarily inaccurate. Recall I like simple. When I look at the old traits attributed to men above—*stoicism, competitiveness, dominance, and aggression* (now considered harmful by that author), I feel they are still alive and well in the world of men in charge of today's world. Perhaps examine also the world of big business and notice what gender is commonly in charge. Do you think a change is needed here too?

Right now, I am appreciating I was guided to include in Part III a Voices of the Goddess, and not a Voices of the masculine counterpart. It makes my job of writing easier . . . and I'm not sure what I would get from a bunch of men not sure of who they are :). And I for one am not particularly interested in promoting more *stoicism, competitiveness, dominance, and aggression* in the world by men or women.

There, I'm glad I got that off my chest. It's part of what I mentioned earlier to keep cleaning out, detoxifying, checking for dust or cobwebs in the corners of all our rooms so we can see clearer, speak clearer, be clearer. It is also possible that I am reaching into a part of my own feminine nature to come up with that assessment. I am often looking at what a balance looks and feels like in our individual components of our masculinity and femininity . . . a job for life I believe.

Did I not mention that this may show up as work sometimes?! The secret is to also experience this as another Bilbo Baggins Adventure . . . and enjoy the ride. Find the fun in it. Explore creativity and levity!

And notice what is showing up for you. What are you discovering about life . . . about your Self?

And now for the Goddesses . . . What do you wish to share with the World? You have center stage now. Everyone is listening to you. I would like to suggest you are at center stage for the rest of your life. Because you are. Now live as such!

Now what?

THE GODDESSES

We are all connected.

This is what I would like to reiterate in my passage for "Voices of the Goddess".

Dear Reader,

One of the most profound understandings that John Mills concludes in this book is "we are all connected".

I could not agree with him more. In my book, *Currency*, I allude to this same concept. I hope you enjoy the following excerpt from my novel, Currency.

Suddenly, Deidre understood a simple truth. All the new-age chatter about everyone being equal, about everyone being connected "as one" had been true all along. She was still marveling over this when another, equally profound awareness hit her — relationships are never with just one person. They are always a mirror. The knowledge that her relationship with any child was a perfect reflection of her relationship with every child left Deidre reeling. Pg 238, Currency ISBN #978-1-800074-191-1

Shanon Harwood

COSMIC GODDESS

A Pleiadian starseed on Earth, I come
From distant stars, a cosmic drum.
My soul yearns for the universe's wonder
But on this planet, my mission lies under.

I am a Cosmic Goddess, ancient and wise,
One of the seven sisters of the celestial skies.
My light shines bright, like the stars in the night
Guiding humanity towards a cosmic flight.

I descend upon this mystical plane,
Where the universe's secrets thunder and rain,
Amongst creatures so different and young,
I learn their secrets and the songs they've sung.

My essence is divine, my magic untold,
In this earthly realm, my presence takes hold.
To help guide humanity to a higher place
Where love knows no bounds and grace meets their face.

For in this universe, love is the key,
A universal language that sets us free.
So I continue on this journey long,
A cosmic traveller, a being of the celestial song.

To share with Earth the magic of the universe,
And help these beings, their divine destiny, traverse.
For I am not of this earthly plane,
My essence is ancient, my wisdom arcane.

But my mission is clear, my purpose strong,
To guide humanity towards where they belong.
Towards a cosmic destiny of love and light,
Guided by the Cosmic Goddess, so bright.

Dayna Catt

For Voices of the Goddess

By

"Ilona Drost"

I want to speak about *feeling*. If you are like me, I was always taught to think, not feel. From early childhood I remember that imagination, feelings, or emotions were unacceptable and not permitted. Only fact was acceptable, and feelings were not fact.

As I moved through my life, thinking became more prominent while feeling took a back seat. Let me clarify what I mean by "feeling". It is not just emotions. It is also sensing, knowing, or having a hunch. When these are fine-tuned, they are a great asset.

Many of us are empaths without knowing it. I didn't know I was one. I thought empaths had special powers and that you were born with a special gift. Many of us have gifts that we don't even realize we have. I know many of us have felt things we cannot explain—maybe a sudden wave that just comes over us or a gut feeling. Often, we don't dare discuss this with someone for fear of being ridiculed. Do you talk yourself out of this feeling, telling yourself that you are just being dramatic or overreacting?

What if you are not overreacting? What if that is your intuition talking to you? What if that is your higher self or a spirit guide reaching out?

Here is my story: I was raised by strongminded, strong-willed Dutch farmers, I married and then divorced. I am an Advanced Care Paramedic and I have been in this line of work for 20 years. I taught myself to think so well that I became a robot. I had created such a hard shell that nothing was coming in or out. I ran on autopilot for so many years without realizing it.

Suddenly I broke, mentally, emotionally, spiritually, psychologically, you name it. I took an 8-month leave of absence from my job. I was in my head so much and lost touch with my inner self to such an extreme.

With both professional and holistic help, and the support of my friends and family and a new spiritual community, I learned to be vulnerable. I started to learn how to feel, slowly, by practicing it every day, with every decision I made. I started reading about shadow work, listening to myself, and truly stepping into my own. I also attended some energy work classes—one of them was the Shaman's Altar, each course divided into four segments, one for each direction (South, West, North and East).

Feeling is a skill. Sensing is a skill. Intuition is a skill. But you have to learn to recognize how a message, a sign, a knowing, feels. You must listen to yourself and try to differentiate between a thought and a feeling, between your head and your heart. Is it a knowing or a telling?

I was very frustrated at first. Again, I was deep in my head trying to be logical about it instead of just being, letting, allowing. I would talk myself out of it, telling myself it was just my imagination. But my shaman teacher said this, and it really rang true for me: Imagination is your higher self talking to you. You should be honored that spirit is speaking to you like that.

Here are some ways to start connecting with your SELF: meditating, yoga, journaling, nature walks, caring for plants, caring for animals, disconnecting from technology, natural grounding foods, sitting in stillness, deep breathing sets, checking in with yourself and ask yourself what you feel versus what you think. Allow yourself to sit with your feelings and learn to label them. Learn to let emotions pass through you, not define you. Take a second, 10 seconds, 5 minutes, an hour, and just feel in the moment. All of this starts with awareness, in small increments.

Learning to feel has really changed my perspective on everyday things. I now have skills I never thought I would have. I am able to feel someone's chakras. I am able to sense things in people. I allow my imagination to tell me what I should know. I allow my guides to be there for me in whichever way they choose. All of this came about after only a year of practicing.

I don't want to say I regret not learning this earlier, because I believe in divine timing, but part of me wishes I would not have wasted so much time *not feeling*. I've often told myself that peace and rest would come later when I'm not so busy. However, that hasn't happened yet. In fact, I am busier now than I have ever been, yet I feel more calm and more at peace now. I knew I resonated with hummingbird, where there is motion in stillness and stillness in motion, one of my teachings in the Altar. And I aim to learn from hummingbird . . . to drink from the sweet nectar of life, and just be.

Ilona

For Voices of the Goddess

By
"Jitka Robinson"

I met John in 2013 during our studies in Yoga and Ayurveda at Kripalu. We became friends instantly. John is one of the kindest, most caring people I've been lucky enough to know and call a good friend. His sense of adventure, hunger for knowledge, enjoyment of life, and brilliant humor, are extraordinary. I think it was two days after we met in Kripalu that I asked John, very seriously, when he is going to write a book to share his stories and wisdom with others. I am beyond excited for this book to be published and so thankful to be friends with a wizard, Shaman John.

. . .

Radiant Heat: A Goddess

Story by "Paige Mills"

I shut my eyes and within a mere moment am pulled back to
Hawaii...simple sunny days spent swimming with dolphins and
working on the farm. Despite my coach's worries with this trip and
how it could impact the precious off-season work, my fastest season
of cross country and my first time earning All-American Honors was
after a summer of training on the Big Island while farming and living
organically.

I rode in the bed of my host mother's truck to the volcano, biting
into avocados while admiring the spectacular view. I was snuggled in
a sleeping bag with Mama Lou the farm pup by my side. My brown
hair was blowing around wildly while her little puppy ears were
flapping fast in the wind behind her face...I couldn't tell who was
more blissed out and I have never felt so at home so far away. I soaked
in every sweet second of this sanctuary I had discovered.

From the moment I met my host mother, who we called Kanoa,
"free one," I felt safe in her presence. Her aura was undeniably bright.
She loved to share stories about her deep connection with the Island
and the healing powers of her South Kona farm. I knew it was no
mistake that our lives intersected.

In addition to harvesting the richest goat milk you will ever taste,
Kanoa actually uses her farm to heal people from around the world
who are battling serious illness. Oh, and let me tell you about her farm!
It's totally off the grid...imagine a rolling hillside paradise, laced with
flowers and palm trees overlooking the bright blue bay...the warm
breeze blows, and the brilliant floral tapestries speak mysterious
messages in the crisp, fresh air. And when the sun sets, millions of
stars paint a portrait so magnificent you are sure to be swept into your
dreams. A nightly bonfire flickers dancing light on the cozy outdoor

kitchen structure, drawing an epic battle of geckos vs spiders hunting bugs in the rafters of the rooftop. To the nature obsessed girl who spent childhood making crystal decorated tree forts in the woods of New Hampshire...this new adventure was a real life dream come true! I couldn't wait to learn from the Island and to learn from this new Mother.

For over an hour we rounded cliffs towering over the pacific, past hillsides rich with wild cattle, and watched as the landscape changed from lush to volcanic. The true beauty of Earth really struck me in this moment. I appreciated the dramatic change of the Earth's surface. It symbolized something greater...the outer surface of life and of people. Both of which can take many different shapes and forms. The view can change from bright green to black rock in a few small steps. But who is to say the new gritty ground isn't as beautiful as the rolling grassy pastures that the cows grazed on? The black volcanic rock tells a different story than the fresh wild meadows. If you listen to her story, her words, you will find value just as beautiful as the flowering hillsides. And if you really open your heart, you may even hear her speak to YOU. Beauty is only skin deep. Whatever her surface appears to be by the naked eye, on the inside, Mother Earth is always glowing...brilliant and hot. Giving us life and feeding her love. Constant love, constant light. You can judge her surface, judge the life that she lets live, but either way she will keep feeding us raw, powerful energy. It's up to us to tap into her heartbeat.

I looked down at my toes and found complete respect for the ground beneath my feet. We stood at a distance in the dark of night, staring at her glowing red heat...proof of how real this Mother we share actually is. We sent our dark energy to Pele, goddess of the volcano, and meditated. Kanoa taught us that if you give Pele your negative thoughts, the thoughts that keep you from thriving, that she will send the energy back to you, new and bright.

I open my eyes, and oh yes...it is very bright! Bright beaming rays of light sting through my eyelids. I squint through my lashes and there it is elevated before me...my broken femur, completely constricted in all of its thigh high casted glory, reflecting the morning sunshine. I take a deep inhale, slowly filling my lungs and close my eyes. Exhaling, I wiggle my toes pressing them against the plaster casting just enough to activate the muscles in my lower leg and stimulate some blood flow. *Strong, fast, fierce. Strong, fast, fierce.* I repeat my affirmations that have accompanied me through many past moments in my running career, good or bad. With another deep breath, I totally relax and send more energy and strength to my knee and leg...I refuse to give in to this limitation.

My father's voice is comforting yet direct on my iPhone speaker as he guides me through my first meditation training session...his optimism is contagious. "Breathe prana into your lungs and through to your broken femur with every conscious inhale. Envision yourself as the strong runner you are, and remember, you are training...pick a new path every day, run it. See the ground before you, witness its beauty. Feel your strength in every stride you take. Breathe. Never forget to breathe...feel prana with every inhale." He tells me that prana, or chi, is the universal life force which embodies not just us humans, but all life on Earth. "Thought precedes form, connect with your prana using positive energy and pure thoughts, and let the healing begin!" He instructs me to devote time every day to my foot exercises, to my "running meditations", and to envision breaking the records I was previously training to surpass.

My dad and I have spent countless hours finding inspiration together...usually through coffee house conversations or hiking the tree-covered trails of Keene. We have built off one another's ideas since I was a child. He is not just my dad. He is a teacher of life and the smartest person I know. He is a family man and a retired Colonel US Army Special Forces with an action-packed life story. He is an orthopedic surgeon and emergency health practitioner who holds additional credentials as a holistic practitioner and certified in the ancient practice of Ayurveda. This fearless yoga teacher doctor dad of ours is your complete balance from the East to the West. He has taught me all that I know about trusting my feet and how to understand and protect myself in an unpredictable world. My dad is the most complex, yet simple example of balance in life...and I am his seed.

When he presented his idea to me about training in my cast, I was immediately bought in and not at all surprised. My dad has been highly trained for survival, and I'll do anything to speed up my recovery. It's no broken femur, but I cross-trained enroute to my collegiate PR in the 5000 meters after rupturing my plantaris tendon...but that's a story for another time. So yes! I love it! I will continue to train, every day in my mind. I will train to run faster than I was before. With dedication and a positive mind, I will be back with my team in no time.

I shut my eyes once more and start training. *Inhale. Exhale...*the warm Hawaii air meets my skin as I revisit this familiar home. Stronger. Faster. With my sneakers laced and hair pulled back in its long ponytail, I step out of my tent to the healing wonderland I have since only seen in my dreams. The bright tapestries whisper secret messages in the breeze, blowing freely through the silent and mysterious air. It feels like one of those mornings Kanoa would talk about with a sparkle in her eye. One of those mornings when you cannot deny that there is a divine presence guiding every step you take. *Deep breath in, and again. Exhale. Looking around, I see no one.*

Stronger. Faster.

The Earth is still, and I run...

By

"Edith Shamrell"

Many years ago, a Catholic nun said to me this sentence: "We all come to this life with a gift, but the purpose of our life is to discover our virtue."

Somehow, this sentence became ingrained in my memory, and now, almost 30 years later, it is still in my mind. I always tried to make sense of it. Over the years I asked myself, "What is my gift, my innate gift, this God-given gift that we are born with?" And most important of all, "What is my virtue?

I came to understand that my gift had always been a certain degree of awareness of what we cannot see with our naked eye. the intangible and invisible world that surrounds us. I had always been aware of other realms of existence other than our 3D World. We Are Spiritual Beings having a human experience. I have always been sensitive to energy, call it spiritual energy from other realms of existence or just the biofield of energy surrounding our physical bodies. I do not practice any religion, but I consider myself a spiritual person. The word virtue by itself already implies a religious connotation. At least that is what I thought for many years, chasing myself out of attending any virtue in this lifetime.

But with the passing of years the meaning of the sentence took another spin for me, and a new meaning came to the surface. I now understand virtue as a talent or quality that we are not born with—as in the case of a gift—but as part of our innate nature, and something we need to cultivate and perfect, like acquiring a new skill that demands hours of practice. This novel approach gave me more giggling room for finding my virtue

After years of pondering this, I became aware that indeed my virtue, as defined in the dictionary, behavioí showing high moíal standards has been affording me the opportunity to learn to accept and embrace my relationship with spirit, my faith in a higher intelligence that animates and guides our lives into discovering tools that get us in tune with our inner compasses. This gut Instinct that we all possess is our birthright, and sometimes it gets shut down by our own mental chatter. It takes a leap of faith to trust our inner compass, and when we do, life gives us rewarding experiences.

This is how I met John Mills, the author of *To Your Health . . . A Work of Art . . . A Work of Fiction*. We both signed up for an Energy Medicine Workshop in Portland Oregon in 2017.

A few months before meeting John I decided to commit myself to trusting my inner voice and intuition, instead of brushing it all out as many times in the past. The universe decided to put me to the test the day I met John at the Energy Medicine workshop.

We were all sitting in a circle and started our introductions when he rejoined the group. Before he even began to introduce himself, I already knew that he was a Shamanic practitioner.

Nothing gave it away; I just intuitively knew. Indeed, he introduced himself as a physician and a shamanic practitioner as well.

After the workshop was finished, I kept having this nudging inner voice suggesting that I ask him for his phone number. This had never happened to me before, and I felt quite uncomfortable.

My mind started brainstorming outcomes.

How could I explain this to him? I was a married woman at the time. What if he thought that I was hitting on him? Because we did not exchange many words during the workshop, how could I explain to him my urge to get his phone number?

Many more questions keep popping up into my head. And the funny thing is that if this same situation had happened four months earlier, I would have brushed it off. But this time I was willing to listen and to act accordingly.

After gathering my courage, and since he was about to leave, I approached him and explained to him that somehow my intuition was telling me to ask for his phone number. He looked at me and to my relief he said, "Sure, I understand, this happens to me all the time." A beautiful friendship started to flourish that day.

After this experience and similar ones, I came to realize that our gift can also give us clues about our virtues; like holding our hand in a gentle way and walking us towards developing feelings of courage, strength, faith, and authenticity; towards helping us to shine our own light in a world in need of as much light as it can get.

Edith Shamrell
Shamanic practitioner and Emotional code certified practitioner.

For Voices of the Goddess

By

"Julie Mills"

My father asked me if I'd be interested in contributing to the part of his book 'Voices of the Goddess,' and considering this an honor, I accepted the invitation without hesitation. In full transparency, my inner procrastinator kicked into high gear with a ferocity that surprised even me. To say I was experiencing resistance is a gross understatement. However, I've arrived at a phase of life where I am exploring what it feels like to look at my own perceived flaws and inhibitions through the lens of compassion, and if compassion is too difficult a lens, I'll attempt the lens of neutrality.

My inner procrastinator has attempted to serve me and protect me in ways I probably will not fully understand. I do not believe that these tendencies, or parts, if you have a predilection for Internal Family Systems (a form of psychotherapy that focuses on a client's internal "parts" and "Self"), originate out of the blue. I believe that my inner procrastinator showed up in my life as a means of protection. I traditionally would feel a sense of disappointment with myself for putting something off, in this instance for six months, but by looking through the lens of compassion I have come to understand that my tendency to procrastinate (especially with creative endeavors such as this) may originate from a place of fear. I immediately feel a softening in my heart when I consider the notion that this driving force in my life to delay creative expressions and pursuits may arise from a false sense of unworthiness and self-doubt. My inner procrastinator is trying to protect me from my belief that I am not worthy. By shining a light on this false sense of unworthiness, I have begun to deconstruct this limiting belief. By deconstructing this limiting belief, that I may not be worthy enough, skilled enough or wise enough to contribute my voice to this book, I have started to construct the new belief that I am worthy, wise and capable of sharing my voice in a meaningful and thoughtful way. Whatever you feel you are not deserving of, I'm here to remind you that you absolutely are.

Our beliefs, many of which live in our subconscious, are potent and powerful, and consequently they will be guiding forces in our lives. My procrastination is a behavior or inclination that I am acutely conscious of, and it has undoubtedly been a driving force in my life. However, I was not conscious of my false sense of unworthiness until I was willing to look closer at the origins of my procrastination. In this sense, procrastination has served as one of my greatest teachers, and it has been a metaphorical portal to shifting my worthiness belief. If a once subconscious belief is unveiled-in my case, "I'm not worthy"-then the power that this limiting belief can generate will become weaker and weaker as it's replaced with the new belief "I am worthy." I have a sense that my tendency to procrastinate may become less frequent as I continue to foster the loving truth that I am worthy of creating whatever it is my heart feels called to share with the world. And so it is for you.

Consider the beliefs you have about yourself that no longer serve you. Is it time to deconstruct these limiting beliefs so that space can be created for the beliefs that serve your highest and most authentic self?

Remember being a child before the age of seven? Maybe those memories are too distant to recall. In that case, take time to witness the way in which a very young child explores and navigates their world. How do they use their eyes, ears, hands, feet, voices and hearts to connect to the present moment? If you observe a healthy, well-adjusted child who is being raised in an atmosphere of love, connection, safety and security, you'll observe a child who unabashedly and decisively connects with the world around them. There's often an inherent sense of trust in the world that children possess because life hasn't proven otherwise, yet this sense of trust tends to erode over time.

As adults, with the passage of time, we often find ourselves becoming more and more reluctant to follow our hearts, take that leap, and boldly step in the direction that inspires and enlivens us. Our hearts carry an intelligence that our minds are incapable of. Our minds are integral to being human and often rooted in survival, but they can often lead us astray as they tend to be misinformed by our societal programming. We often start to live trapped in the confines of the conditioning that our society so dutifully bestows upon us, at the cost of a truly meaningful and self-actualized life.

Pay attention to those whispers from your heart that are softly urging you to go in a different direction. The mind will likely try to interject and provide you with a litany of reasons as to why you shouldn't follow your heart. A dissonance can often arise between the heart and the mind, and this inharmonious relationship can lead to tension and confusion on one end of the spectrum, and pain, suffering and anguish on the other. Try to have appreciation for your mind's attempts at interference, as its main objective is to keep you safe. Politely deflect the mind's misinformed conjurings and tune into the frequency of your heart and where it is trying to guide you.

Don't be afraid to take steady, consistent and sometimes bold and courageous steps in the direction of your dreams. If the notion of stepping in the direction of your dreams seems too daunting right now, take a single step toward something that enlivens you. Your heart is speaking to you when you are engaged in an experience that feels expansive, joyous, energizing, and profoundly meaningful. Trust those emanations. Small, incremental steps in the direction of that thing that generates a visceral sense of joy within you will unequivocally lead you in the direction of a more inspired and purposeful life. In every event or opportunity that arises, connect to the visceral intelligence of your heart. It will always inform you as to whether or not something is in alignment with your highest good, or not.

One could create a compelling argument that presence is integral to connecting with your heart intelligence. What feels true for me is that each breath is also integral to connecting with one's heart intelligence. One begets another. Each and every moment is the most essential moment. Each and every breath is the most essential breath.

Once the moment is gone, once you've exhaled, you're gifted with yet another moment and another inhalation. Instead of considering each moment as a means to another moment, each breath as a means to another breath, consider each moment and each breath as an opportunity for connection with your heart intelligence. I have come to realize that each breath taken is a bridge between mind and heart. Each breath serves as a bridge between cognition and embodied awareness.

Embodied awareness is a practice that we all have access to. By attuning to the sensations in our bodies we can gain awareness relative to our current emotional, physical, or mental states. Embodied awareness is an essential step in attuning to heart intelligence. Feeling your emotions fully is one aspect of embodied awareness.

Resist the temptation to avoid, escape, numb, deflect or distract yourself from what is arising. Feeling your emotions fully will allow you to process and transmute them.

Refusing to feel your emotions fully is an invitation for suffering, emotional blockages, and ultimately a life unfulfilled and uninspired.

I started to integrate this concept into my life several years ago, and this simple act has been transformational in my life. I used to try to escape from uncomfortable feelings and emotions by distracting myself with the many things available to us humans (the list is endless). I now use emotional or physical pain as an opportunity to lean into discomfort by tuning into my body, noticing the sensations that are present, and being with what arises while simultaneously breathing into the spaces that feel tense and constricted. I visualize an inhalation of peace and love and an exhalation of distress and pain. I try to untether any specific sensations in my body from any thoughts conjured in my mind. The mind can often be rooted in fear, anxiety, judgment, and thoughts about the past and future. By attuning to the sensations of the body while experiencing a heightened emotion and detaching from any associated thoughts that may be perpetuating the emotion, the body innately wants to allow the emotion to pass.

This practice takes repetition. LOTS of repetition. I constantly default to old patterning, multiple times a day, and these are the instances when I reach for the "quick fix." These are the instances when I turn away from embodied awareness and my heart intelligence. However, every day I'm confronted with opportunities to feel my emotions deeply and I choose to embrace them instead of pushing them away and abandoning them.

To fully integrate into my body I take a deep breath, I place one hand over my heart and the other hand on my belly, and as I exhale I shift from noticing my thoughts to observing the sensations within my body. I notice the warmth that is generated between my hand and my chest. I notice the subtle sensation of each heartbeat that is detected by my hand. I hear the voice of my heart intelligence. I notice the rise and fall of my ribcage as my lungs inhale and exhale. I feel the activation of my solar plexus, the chakra that governs our sense of confidence, assertiveness, and self-esteem. I feel connected. I feel embodied. I feel present. I feel grateful.

Every time I use this exercise when confronted with an unpleasant emotion or sensation, which can often arise when my inner procrastinator takes center stage, it doesn't take long before I can tap into an internal atmosphere of love, connection, safety and security. This is the condition that allows my inner procrastinator to quietly exit stage left. This is where true self-empowerment lies. My desire is for all humans to live in an internal AND external atmosphere of love, connection, safety and security. I believe it starts on an individual level, and if that is actualized, it has the potential to expand to the level of family, community, and globe. Let us start with a simple inhale and exhale.

Thank you, dad, for inviting my voice to be a part of your inspiring and transformational message.

Love, Julie

For Voices of the Goddess

By
"Madison Mills"

The other day I visited the ocean. I was eager to get there all day, as it was the only place I wanted to be. I felt like I needed to be there, like something was pulling me there. It was getting dark but that didn't matter to me. I jumped in and felt welcomed by whatever was out there. I love the ocean. It is overwhelmingly alluring. I told my Dad about my experience which inspired him to write the poem below.

With My Feet In The Sand

It was just after sunset
I was standing on the shore
at Salt Pond Beach
Gentle waves caressing my feet
And then she spoke to me

With the rhythm of her heartbeat
Matching mine
We shared this moment of deep sensing
and mutual understanding
My feet buried in the sand feeling her pulse

She opened a door for me

A doorway into my Soul
And I knew in that moment
What steps I was to take
As Gaia took my hand
And walked with me
With the Spirit of Kaua'i

Madison

For Voices of the Goddess

By

"Alana N Agustin"

(Alana offered two voices, both touch the heart, so both were included)

You are an amazing strong beautiful human being. Your body is a wonderful vessel that has already taken you, and will continue taking you, through so much in life. Care for her, love her, appreciate her, and know that you already are all the little things that make her special to you that you may not even see. After many years of turbulence and trauma I realized that my greatest gift to you and to myself was to say, *"Don't get upset about anything you can't change."*

So if your sadness or your madness can't change the situation—and it rarely can—then just let it go. Set that boundary for yourself, say no more, and say yes to yourself more. Live in your truth. That's all that matters. Be your own biggest fan and accept nothing less from the people that you share your air with.

Or you can use my life-changing story as inspiration . . .

In May of 2015 I was 29 years old. My father passed just 1 month shy of my youngest Daughter, Dakota's, first birthday, and a few months shy of his 51st birthday. I never in a million years thought that for 2 years in my 20s I would be watching a parent pass and spending my time caring for him in my home. It was such a challenging time where things seemed to pile up on top of each other so terribly. I felt I was drowning in bills, emotions, and exhaustion. But we made it through those very hard 2 years. That experience helped me realize that I could manage any stress I encounter or achieve any goal I set.

Being an advocate for my Dad's health made me stronger, as I had to stand up for what he wanted even when others didn't agree with him or with me.

Through this experience I learned a lot about myself through advocating for him. I learned to appreciate every moment and every breath shared with the ones we love, and to love and care for ourselves more. Women are natural caregivers, mothers, lovers, sisters and daughters. Too often we forget that we must take the time to give ourselves care, to love ourselves, and to make ourselves a priority. We must learn to say *YOU ARE WORTH IT, EVERY MINUTE OF YOUR LIFE!* Honor yourself and know that every bad minute or hard minute of life has its season and will change and shift. Don't let yourself sit in a season that isn't serving you. Make the move, take the trip, change the job, get therapy if you need it, do it all, because we all never know when our season is up.

Mahalo Nui Loa,

Alana N Agustin
Echelon Beauty Kauai

For Voices of the Goddess

By
"Kazumi Sakurai"

I found a sign in a Shinto temple in Japan that said, "Illness is a time to look back on the mistakes you've made" 病気とは反省する時 Sickness or trouble in life gives us a chance to reflect ourselves. If we can use this chance, we can understand ourselves better. Our body, hidden stress, untreated desires, how we think, patterns...myself. We don't know anything, but we think we know. When the chances are here, we get panic, depressed, and feel pain physically and mentally. We start seeking help, go to see Doctor, search, read books, talk to specialist, change the diet, start exercises, look back on our past, collecting information to find some answers to better understand myself.

It is painful to look at truth, but without doing it, life will not send us chance to heal.

We cannot avoid this, but it is still really hard to face each moment completely and still be true to myself. Many times I want to be numb, zoning into movies, internet, working hard, alcohol. Even with something that sounds healthy like meditation and exercises could be just a type of escape. We might be doing it since we are little, so it is hard to see what we are doing to numb ourselves, not facing the truth. Then the kind universe will give us to realize that we are doing something wrong.

Health is owning complete responsibility for one's life. We can still ask for help, but we need to know that true healing happens by us when we are fully committed and ready. That's what I think of seeking health and happiness in this moment of my life.

Kazumi

For Voices of the Goddess

By

"Dr. Alanna Golden"

I feel so honored to participate in John's book which is a beautiful contribution for humankind. It's time to awaken and to connect deeper within ourselves.

It's important to raise the perception of our own physical temple and to get more knowledge about how to take care of our own bodies. That's an invitation at the same time to be open to more magic and beauty in our paths. When we are open to discover more about our own nature, we can let go and let flow the crystal energies, and transformation happens.

I have been dedicating my life in sharing the Path of Beauty and Shamanism through our daily actions. This planetary journey is very generous with a great life and many blessings. As part of our contribution with humanity we want to produce more books, teach with healing sound, participate in ceremonies, sacred dances, meditations, rituals, natural therapies, amazing journeys at the sacred spots, ancient teachings, and much more.

Meditation is one of the keys in the path of self-realization, as I share in my book *The Pilgrim*, *"it is in the simplicity of the moment with an open heart that spiritual peace is found. By journeying deep into our self do we realize the greatness and the worthiness of our value."*

We understand how beautiful and unique we are. *"Once we embark on the path of Being, we assume another view of the World, since we understand it is we who construct it."* The Divine essence of every Self is the reflection of the beauty that exists within the Universe.

It is up to us to build together a New World with more peace, beauty and universal love. Embracing you all from Cusco to connect heart with heart.

We are all one.

Dra Evelyn Guimaraes del Paiva –
Dr. Alanna Golden

For Voices of the Goddess

By

"Leilani Levesque"

Inner Goddess

Listen to yourself
Quiet the mind and observe
By being curious we can ask the questions
And the answers will come
Working in the energetic creates the physical world
with more ease

Be grateful, and feel it
See all you have
This builds abundance

Our relationships, connections, and
shared experiences and adventures are our treasures

Ground out into the earth and release all your pain
Let your inner light shine surrounding your body and filling your
spirit
We are here to heal and help heal
Do not blame others. It is a waste of time
Ask what can I do? What am I tolerating?
What do I need to change?

All the answers are within us.
We just need to be clear enough to listen.

. . .

Leilani Levesque

Well, the Goddesses have spoken, at least all of them up until now. I sense more will come in later for inclusion in this book or a later one. I sense there are many Goddesses who wish to speak. I will declare Part III complete at this time.

This brings me to the question at this point, *"Why didn't the ones speak who said they wanted to, who were enthusiastic about the idea and in contributing their voices?"* . . . *even after I sent out reminders more than once, and most were still interested, not all, but most.*

And there was an international stage of women, all friends and people I know personally who were willing to participate. Their countries of origin included Spain, India, Japan, Canada, Poland, Philippines, Peru, Ecuador, Brazil, England, Czech Republic, and the United States.

This participation or not gave me the opportunity to really consider why this was so. I explained to all of them this was an opportunity for each to express anything they wished to say to the whole world without editing, without restriction. It was intended to be from each Goddess's heart exactly what she wanted to say. I expressed my intention that I was going for a global audience, that I eventually saw many in the whole world reading this. And I saw all this as the design of something much beyond me that simply wanted to be expressed through me through this book. I explained all this earlier.

What this offered me was another opportunity to walk my talk. I simply got to see that the season wasn't right for everyone to speak at this time but that it was perfect for the ones who did speak at this time. That simple! It was not about what I wanted but about what was to be at this time. This was very important to acknowledge—for me and for every reader. There was no need for disappointment, make wrong, be critical of anything. I have in fact been there more times than I can count . . . the one who didn't get something done on time when it was requested of me. Not completing something agreed to means not completing something agreed to. It's that simple. Leave the story out unless it serves everyone to tell it. That was my lesson. This can be a lesson for us all.

A first interpretation could be: *I am afraid to speak to the world, I am not good enough to speak to the world, why would the world want to hear anything from me, I'm too busy, I don't have time for this, why did I agree to do this in the first place, and on and on and on* . . . More of the Monkey Mind, remember? All of those reasons would describe me at one time or another. And none of those reasons matter, except perhaps to the person speaking them, and then it is up to only that person as to how their interpretation shows up in their life.

What I was really hoping for was that everyone would play, all would contribute something, because I believed and still do, that the words written from the heart of every woman (Goddess) would be important to share with the whole world.

On the other hand, I will acknowledge that some did answer the call this time around and those are the words shared above. Each contributed such a uniquely beautiful part of their story. I can only imagine what a world of women would say to the world as they tap into their heart energy and creative abilities. Stay tuned. More is to come :)

The more to come includes my invitation to each of you—to every woman on the planet—to dive deeply into your heart of hearts and find words that would benefit the world we live in, words that would make a difference to Mother Earth and all her beings, and then speak them in any way you choose to whomever you choose.

Perhaps begin slowly in small bites, but expand to big slices (read that as big ideas), keeping in mind two things we already spoke of . . . remember the pebble thrown into the pond creating ripples going out into the universe in all directions, and to DREAM BIG.

What do you wish to send out into the universe . . . forever? What are you Dreaming now?

Thank you all for your willingness to speak as the Goddesses you are—it is your birthright as I see it—and thank you for the inevitable changes each of you will bring to our World.

We will do this again sometime soon.

John Mills

APPENDIX A

OFFICE HANDOUTS

These handouts were designed by me out of what I viewed as a series of general concerns of many of my patients over the years. Since I have always embraced a Holistic philosophy—looking at the whole person—I was always willing to engage with my patients comprehensively whenever possible as to their life concerns and their lifestyles. A variety of approaches proved of value and unique to each patient's needs and interests. Here then follows those handouts, my patients often opting to take all of them when offered in hard copy form in my office. Each of you readers may decide which is of value to you personally and ignore the rest.

HEALTHY LIFESTYLE AND HEALING

We all have an automatic Lifestyle granted us by being born a human being. What we do with this life—our style of living life—is our choice after we become adults. Those choices may largely be affected by the life we experienced as children entrusted to the care of others. Our choices for living life well, or not, influence our ability to do well or heal well or not. To examine one's lifestyle and make choices for a life lived well can be a challenge to us all at times. Our childhood experiences play a great role in this. Nevertheless, the more aware and proficient we become at guiding our life on this path helps determine the quality of our life. This path naturally spills over into those around us—our family and friends, our work and play environment, and the community with which we engage over all our years.

Lifestyle then becomes about the kind of person we are, the many diverse experiences we bring to our lives, the friends we choose, our relationships with family and friends, our work, our play, our activities, and whether we are consciously aware of our own lives as we grow and the decisions we make at every step of the way. That's a lot to think about. Most of us however fall onto a certain path and one thing leads to another often unconsciously or without awareness. Life just happens to us. It doesn't have to, but it often shows up like this for many. What is important at any time is to see if we are on a runaway train and want to get off before it crashes, or are we happy with the way our life is going? This is the short course—Lifestyle 101.

The graduate level is us doing our life day by day, adjusting every day as we deem necessary, perhaps with short-range and long-range plans, with a certain notion of ways to stay healthy and fit and enjoy the journey. There are always clues along the way so staying alert and vigilant and open helps.

The important part is to notice we have some say in the course our life takes, and to affect these course changes when we feel ready. Many of us don't realize we get a vote in how our life looks until we do. That's when Lifestyle becomes a matter of real importance and direction. Who are friends are, what we eat, where we work and spend our leisure time all play a role. These things often just happen to us when suddenly we notice things aren't working out so well. That's usually what it takes for us to become more vigilant of our own life— when it really starts to matter to us. Often this happens because of major upsets or breakdowns or breakups in our life. Relationships ending or very troubled, major illness or injury occurring to us or our loved ones, and trauma and tragedies too numerous to identify, are often sufficient to cause most of us to take a different and deeper look at how we are living our life.

This page is not about fixing your life. It is about taking closer notice of your life, and if changes are indicated then bringing them about for your betterment. As many things as you can think of, can affect your lifestyle and therefore your health. Choice of place to live, go to school, work, friends, mate, diet, activities, life experiences, are all on the table. Becoming more resilient and self-reliant are big advantages. This can become a lifetime study and worth it.

John Mills MD

DIET AND NUTRITION

It is my intention to make simple some of the most important things toward creating good health and healing on the planet for humans. Since we are all blessed with consciousness and a will, we need to put this to good use for the choices we make. A healthy person in mind and body can remain this way his or her entire life with some added awareness and mindfulness in thought and deed.

What we eat, how we eat, when we eat plays a significant role. If I suggested we eat healthy most of the time, most of us know what that means. Doing it is another matter. I will sum up my experience over a lifetime that offers up some healthy suggestions and each of us can take it from there. The rewards will become obvious.

Eat fresh fruits and vegetables, organic or locally grown without pesticides is best, and seasonally when available—if it's grown where you live in that season, that's a good choice. Eat fruits and veggies of all colors, the so-called rainbow diet, containing many phytonutrients. Green leafy vegetables and cruciferous vegetables like broccoli, cauliflower, bok choy, kale, collard greens, brussels sprouts, to name a few. Explore and become creative in your choices and recipes.

Proteins in the form of meats, beans, nuts, in modest amounts are necessary for the amino acids they contain—cellular building blocks. Healthy fats and oils are good for you—medium chain triglycerides, coconut oil, ghee (clarified butter) and butter made from grass fed cattle (if you do dairy in any form), while any nut milks that you like are good for non-dairy diets. Fish oils are good for you too. Study vitamin and mineral and other supplements as you make your decisions.

Stay away from—for the most part—junk food, processed white sugar and white flour products, canned, boxed, and processed foods, chemicals, and eating too much at one sitting. Avoid grazing—eating small amounts all day long. Your digestive system needs rest between meals. Don't eat before bedtime and try not to eat any later than 6 or 7 in the evening. The stomach should be done digesting and empty before you go to sleep. That's when the repair work on your body happens and if the energy is being spent on digestion it is diverting it from repair work.

Don't eat when emotionally upset or angry. Don't eat with the TV on or while monitoring any other electronic devices—and in fact, unless part of your work, keep electronics at a minimum in your life. Always think of your body as a sacred temple, and the care you render it will serve you well for your entire lifetime. Disease and disability are not necessary. They are products of not making good choices in our life over and over again. Keeping our bodies light, fit, flexible, happy, joyful, and mobile, our whole lifetime is key. Not only do the foods we eat affect our health, but the thoughts we think and the deeds we do also affect our health, as well as our recovery from any illness or injury. Choose to make this a lifetime study. You and your family are worth it.

John Mills MD

SELF-CLEANSING AND DETOXIFICATION

We are constantly exposed to toxins in our daily life and increasingly so with every passing year. In fact, it can be accurately stated that we live in a virtual sea of toxicity via the air we breathe, the food we eat, the water we drink (and swim in), and the many choices we make every day that appear innocent but are not. We now know that this is adversely affecting our health, our ability to recover from illness and injury, and potentially devastating effects await future generations if we do not take a stand and take action on reversing this.

The first and most important thing we can do is attend to the toxicity in our own bodies and begin to manifest a healthy body and mind and quality of life. How do we best accomplish this? First it is important to become aware of it, and then to do something about it. And be ever mindful that thoughts and feelings can be toxic also and can affect our health adversely. Help flush out toxins by drinking lots of pure water and by having healthy thoughts.

The toxins that fill our bodies are a product of our so-called advanced civilization and our diets and lifestyle. We ingest many toxic chemicals in the food we eat and the water we drink. Simplifying and purifying our diets is a good beginning. Many of us have awakened to the importance of this. Many of us have not. It is important to eat a clean healthy diet that is more natural and therefore supports our body's health and immune system. Nature is your partner. Eat naturally. Fresh fruits and vegetables are the mainstay of healthy eating. Processed foods lack live cells, enzymes, and nutrients that are essential to nourishing our bodies.

Proteins are essential also—the so-called essential amino acids are from sources outside our bodies and are called essential because they are. If we eat meat, it should be from a healthy source, including grass fed, as well as knowing of the care and respect the animals receive from meadow to table. If we choose not to eat meat, there are many healthy sources of protein that can be found in nuts, beans, legumes, and a variety of other sources. Whole grains, organically grown, or locally grown without pesticides, are important. Processed white sugar and white flour are considered toxins in some cultures. Avoid all processed foods whenever possible.

So, in addition to eating quality, clean and naturally occurring foods, be mindful of all the chemicals that accompany that which we call food but is not. Read the labels, eat fresh whenever possible, shop the perimeter of the grocery store where the fresh stuff hangs out and skip canned and boxed stuff in the center isles, or grow you own at home when possible.

As for the toxins already polluting our bodies, our cells, our very DNA, begin a cleanse of your choosing. Intermittent fasting is one way. Look into the many self-cleanse programs now offered and find one that calls to you. I am available to discuss this in detail if desired. It is very important to keep our system clean, operating smoothly, and to periodically take out the garbage as it builds up. This is not just a good idea. It is essential to creating good health and vitality.

John Mills MD

WEIGHT MANAGEMENT

This is only for those who are interested in managing their weight. Whatever your weight, it is your state of health and your desire to gain or lose weight that is important, perhaps allowing your perceived state of health to be your guiding principle. There are Sumo wrestlers in Japan who are naturally big, with excess body fat in many. One of these wrestlers has his students attack him as part of their training, and they bounce off his energy field never able to make physical contact with him—perhaps a very healthy individual.

For many, being overweight or underweight is a sign of ill health or predicts ill health to follow. This can be viewed from a variety of perspectives and there are a number of ways to return to what you see as your desired optimal weight. Often it is not a simple formula like eating less or exercising more that takes the pounds off if you are overweight. Both can be beneficial for some. There is more to the story. Not just quantity of food, but quality of food, when you eat, under what circumstances, emotional state, family history and family health, relationships, work environment and on and on, are to be taken into consideration on a case-by-case basis.

"I've always been heavy," or "It runs in my family," are explanations offered by some of those who are unsuccessful in their weight loss programs. But ask yourself if you are one of these, does it serve you? There are always ways one can address this issue even when there is a perceived and self-constructed wall in the way. There is also the metabolic explanation of hormonal influences. And for those who see (or not) the building on of extra layers as an insulating protection against deep emotional wounds, hurts, adverse childhood experiences, societal pressures, this is yet another interpretation.

There is also the reliance on comfort foods in our often-stressful life on a daily basis to soothe life's upsets or chronic anxiety. There is also the built-in reasoning of not participating more fully in many of life's activities that require a strong, fluid, lighter body to participate. Remember this conversation on weight management is not for those who feel healthy, well balanced, and happy with the way their life is. The list can go on and on. There Is no right or wrong way to show up in life. It is your call entirely, and your decision to do something about it or not.

There are far too many options, and way too much advice on how YOU should do it. Don't pay attention to any of it! But do educate yourself and attune to your inner guidance and align with your own inner program for achieving health and wellbeing. Your optimal weight will soon fall into line with your vision for what you desire for your SELF. This is all related to your body's blueprint for what is needed for optimal healthy living. Just clear out all that is in the way and this process becomes natural. Consider creating this without struggle. Consider this can be done with effortless ease. It just takes a willingness to explore your Self, to deepen the inquiry, to discover what is in the way and then shed it. Perhaps see that which you wish to create for your Self NOW before it manifests. I'm happy to discuss this further with anyone so interested.

John Mills MD

EXERCISE

For those of you who exercise regularly, you already know the value. What you may not be aware of is it is important to exercise throughout your entire life no matter your age. For those of you who haven't made exercise a regular part of your life, consider doing so, as it adds immeasurably to the quality of your life. This has been stated and proven over and over again for many years. That exercise keeps you youthful, fit, and healthy is beyond question. We keep refining the importance of exercise and for those who pay attention there are many benefits.

Commonly we consider exercise as a physical thing, which is very important by the way—it is a very physical thing. Longevity and quality of life are clearly a result of attending to the body in the many forms of movement available. Maintaining strength and flexibility your entire life is a key ingredient to good health. The body wants to move and be challenged. You pick the way you accomplish this. Will most of you agree that many of us humans have largely become less active and more sedentary over the years, especially as we age, and even so for our children?

Exercise also applies to our mind. It too needs exercise and development throughout our whole life. How many of us engage in the passive form of using our mind—like TV, cell phone use, social media? How many of us are still studying something, anything, to expand our mind, our experience of life, our level of awareness, considering our purpose in life, and then becoming active in fulfilling it? How many of us are practicing imagination and dream fulfillment?

There is much evidence that just putting our awareness on anything we wish to change, heal from, grow into, become, brings the necessary energy to that vision and begins accomplishing it for us. If we consider that our very thoughts are a form of energy—and they are—just thinking about and perhaps visualizing the outcome we desire begins that transformation. Similarly, if we have anything blocking that vision, that intention, that energy, it takes more work to discover it and remove it, however it is still doable. The underlying message here: Choose your thoughts wisely.

Exercising your experience of fun, joy, play, relaxation, leisure time wisely utilized, takes first awareness that it is possible, and then practice seeing if we can create more of it, to balance out other areas of our life, all contributing to our overall sense of happiness and wellbeing. This is not a matter of wondering if it is possible. It is a matter of knowing it is possible and then discovering the ways it can be experienced in our life. Who are we talking to, or what are we reading or listening to, in the pursuit of these experiences? Consider many of us are busy paying attention to the lives and dramas of others while ignoring our Selves in the process.

Where and how would we like to bring more exercise to our life? Take a moment to write this down to make it a little bit more real in your life? . . . like a to-do list for creating extraordinary in your life, and then begin it.

John Mills MD

STRESS AND INFLAMMATION

Stress and inflammation are included together here because they are related. How many of you are aware of this? Stress has become almost a universal experience in the modern world, and this stress has become chronic. It was not a chronic experience for our hunter-gatherer ancestors who experienced stress as a now and then experience based upon what was happening in their immediate lives in the moment. It is also not the experience of certain indigenous populations living in the so-called blue zones on the planet today where the people live calmly in balance with nature, eating fresh food from the land and the sea, and where high blood pressure, heart disease and cancer are virtually unknown.

Modern humans wake up with stress, spend most of their days under stress, and then go to sleep feeling stress. That is to say that the once in a while flight or fight experience has now become a chronic thing. Our adreno-corticoids are constantly flooding our systems with this flight or fight hormone, very useful to rev up the system to save our lives when to flee or stand and fight were the only two options to an immediate threat. This has now been transferred to an all day, every day stressful experience that is harming us. Our adrenal glands are becoming depleted. Chronic stress—real or imagined—is one of the main causes of inflammation in the body. And inflammation is one of the main causes of cancer and heart disease worldwide.

It has been known for some time that cancer and heart disease are the two main causes of death for us humans worldwide. Both diseases kill men and women equally and account for half the deaths in the world. That is astounding. And it is especially astounding when we connect the dots and note that chronic inflammation contributes greatly to these conditions, and chronic stress contributes greatly to chronic inflammation. In other words, all these deaths are mostly preventable by wise diet and lifestyle choices. You can draw your own conclusions but at least give this notion consideration. Put this knowing into practice and it may just save your life. It may even allow you a much better quality of life and living.

So, we can approach this problem in one way—at the diet and lifestyle level—or we can move to the stress level and just learn to relate to our stresses in life in a healthier way. Just change your perspective and maybe your perception of stress. Stress can be a teacher, even a friend here to inform us of the importance of making better choices. And we can adopt ways to still and calm ourselves, through well-known activities such as exercise, Yoga, breathwork, biofeedback, meditation, Nature walks, creative endeavors of our choice that serve to relax us, to name a few. It is probably important to be willing to learn what stress is saying to us. In changing our perspective, in surrendering to the message stress is sending us, we can then take a more responsible and healthier approach to our so-called stressful experience. We can relate to it differently. We can manage it differently. And sometimes we can simply walk away from it and say *No* to it, *I'm not playing*. We can choose another less stressful path. What do you think?

John Mills MD

PAIN

It has been stated many times: Pain is part of life. It is also probably a true statement that every human being who has ever walked this earth has experienced pain in some form at one time or another. We've all heard that pain is a learning experience—like if we put our hand in a flame it will get burned and cause pain. This teaches us not to put our hand in a flame again.

And emotional or mental pain is another example, less obvious perhaps but with the same message—whatever it was that caused the experience of mental or emotional pain provides us an opportunity to be more mindful of what caused the pain and perhaps teaches us to interact with the experience in a way that causes us less or no pain in the future. Does this make sense?

My take on this is that some of us are slow learners, myself included. It is true that we all have accidents at times that produce a painful outcome, and sometimes a lasting disability and chronic pain. We will come to *lasting and chronic* below, as these may be addressed in another domain.

There are many interpretations of why pain is in our lives: as a teacher, as a learning experience, as a blocked flow of energy in our body, as a karmic debt being paid, or an ancestral imprint. But can we experience pain as a friend, embrace it? It has been said, *what we resist persists.*

In its simplest form pain is just another sensation in the body, but because it is not a pleasant sensation, we don't want it. We resist it. What would happen if we worked with it, if we communicated with it, asked the pain why it is in our life and what would it take for it to leave. I already see your eyes rolling, wondering if I'm crazy. Perhaps, but pretend I'm not. I've done this successfully with myself and even with some of my patients. It has been part of my journey of Self-discovery and then something to share since pain is such a universal phenomenon. And then some of us just need to carry pain in our life until we don't anymore, part of our journey perhaps.

If we allow that pain is just another sensation in our system—our physical, mental, emotional body—that has a purpose, not good or bad, just an experience to work with, perhaps this leaves us more empowered to engage successfully with it. I don't know. I'm just suggesting we consider this. I have tried this in the test tube called my body and discovered things of value that I wouldn't have if I were not willing to look deeper into the experience. When we experience love and joy, we desire more of that. When we experience pain, we want less of that. In the illusion that life has been called by the wise ones it has been said that it is not the goodness or badness that we assign something but the experience itself that matters. What can we learn from the experience?

I will suggest that each of us decide for ourselves what the experience our pain has to offer us. I have some experience with this, and the deeper I look, the more I learn about my life and the choices I have made—not good or bad ones, just choices, each with their own outcomes and experiences. Perhaps you wish to take a deeper look and see what you discover.

John Mills MD

FUN, PLAY, JOY, LAUGHTER, LEVITY

Any conversation on achieving health and wellbeing would be incomplete if the above were not included in the conversation. For those of us who experience these qualities regularly in our lives, we know the importance of it. In my role as a physician over the years I have observed that these qualities when experienced regularly have much to do with the generation of a healthy life experience, and this contributes to health and longevity. It's like a law of Nature. But discover this for yourself by practicing it. There is barely any effort involved. Some of you may have even heard there is more effort expended in the work our facial muscles do to frown than to smile.

How often do we smile? What makes us smile? Who makes us smile? These are worthwhile questions and shine a light on the path our life is taking. How many of you were drawn to this title when looking over the one-page handouts I've designed? These words seem to just call to many of us, and the experiences behind them that all of us can associate with, even if infrequently. These messages, these feelings of happiness and joy speak to every cell in our body. They take part in the experience, and this encourages optimal performance from each of them. This is not just my opinion. I am not the only one to have said this. We can communicate with all parts of our body consciously anytime. This is a knowing available to all of us but even research has discovered this. Play with this notion and see what shows up for you :). Or just play and see what shows up.

Our physiology plays a role too. Have you heard of the science of Neuro-Linguistic Programing— known as NLP? There is a reason depressed people are always looking down. Do an experiment: Look up at the sky and then try to feel depressed. Even if you are feeling depressed over something really depressing, look up and hold you gaze upward and try to feel depressed. What happens? For me, I start laughing when I do this. Change your physiology, change your mood.

Talk to your body, and all its parts, and all your cells, about good things, happy things, healing things, and see what the response is. And no, you don't have to do this out loud :). It's the thought and the intention behind it that counts.

How many of you pay attention to the faces of people you pass or see on the street, or even meet? Notice what's there. Is there a sense of levity or lightness? Is there a sense of life's-not- working- out-well and perhaps anxiety or depression, or a pained look? Notice how this communicates to you—how does each expression affect how you feel. Any difference? You see this is a power we each hold, to influence the lives of others positively or negatively.

Next notice children at play, at home, on a playground or a swimming pool, or at the beach, (without the adults controlling every moment with the No's and the Don't do that's). Doesn't it make you feel joyful? Perhaps not, if your own childhood was not that, if it was filled with No's and Don't's. You can change this at any time. Change your physiology, change your mood. Begin playing and laughing now. It will be fun. And levity, lightness, and enlightenment are all related.

John Mills MD

BALANCE

In the ancient wisdom teachings of Ayurveda, to bring oneself into balance brings about self- healing—it allows all dis-ease to leave the body, be it physical, mental, or emotional. This wisdom comes from a science thousands of years old and is still practiced today throughout the world. Its origins stem from ancient Hindu writings. This is not dissimilar from ancient traditional Chinese Medicine as both sciences share the same roots and are based upon observances of Nature and the natural world. Shamanism also speaks of the importance of bringing oneself into Ayni—into balance, into reciprocity, with the universe, into alignment with Nature and all that is. That to do so brings about a dissolution of all that is no longer needed, and which holds us back on our journeys to Self-discovery and to Selfhood.

The next obvious question is how does one attain balance? Perhaps not so obvious but very important to explore. The immediate answer is it depends. It depends upon each one of us and where we are out of balance and what we can do to reestablish balance, perhaps easier stated than done. Try a balance pose from Yoga, like Vrksasana (tree). It may carry over into your life.

Just by bringing awareness to this quality of balance in your life, you begin the process of finding balance. For starters, just look. What do you see that is out of balance? Pick the obvious stuff first, and the less than obvious stuff will become more apparent. It is after-all a practice, like life itself, if desiring to practice life artfully.

For me, the obvious stuff includes but is not limited to what I invite into my daily life, some by choice, but most unconsciously. As

Ayurveda teaches us, it is the body's natural propensity to go out of balance even when in balance. One must be mindful of the subtle variations of thoughts and actions—read that as lifestyle—that create imbalances and then catch these imbalances before they become disease. Studying the basics of Ayurveda is a good place to learn more about this science and how your life may benefit from it. How do we balance our diet, our workday, our exercise and rest, our relationships, our giving and receiving, our masculine and feminine aspects, our levels of life participation and enjoyment, our goals with the consideration of our families and loved ones? This will be different for each and every one of us to discover.

We are all unique.

So when we look, what do we see that is out of balance? Next, we can ask our Selves, what our Self sees is out of balance, what does it feel is out of balance? There will be responses. Learn to trust these. I have been down this road and have learned to trust these responses, these intuitive hits that are always available to us when we ask. Then it may take some Tapas, some fire, some discipline, to act on our intuition to restore balance—again, easier said than done—but it's a beginning. Once the inquiry has begun, it can open the door to more Self-discovery and Balance.

Start with finding stillness, listening, looking deeply, being with Nature, and opening to Self. There will be clues. You will feel them. Then Act. Then Be-come in Balance.

John Mills MD

APPENDIX B

BOOKS TO GROW BY

don Miguel Ruiz (MD, Surgeon, Shaman)
The Four Agreements Voice of KnowledgeThe Mastery of Love

don Oscar Miro-Quesada (Maestro Curandero, Psychologist,
Shaman)
Lessons in Courage

Alberto Villoldo (PhD, Medical Anthropologist, Shaman)
Healer, Shaman, Sage
The Four Insights
Grow A New Body

Carl Greer (Jungian Psychologist, Shaman)
Change Your Story, Change Your Life

Caroline Myss
Anatomy of Spirit
Sacred ContractsArchetypes

Donna Eden
Energy Medicine
Energy Medicine for Women

Lauren Walker
Energy Medicine Yoga

Michael Singer
The Untethered Soul

Deepak Chopra (MD, Ayurveda, Holistic Practitioner)
The Seven Spiritual Laws of Success (and many more)

Vasant Lad (Ayurvedic Physician, One of my Teachers)
Any books by Dr Lad, a number on natural medicines for home use
See the movie about his life on Neflix—The Doctor From India

Kulreet Chaudhary, MD and Ayurvedic Physician at Tamil Nadu,
India
Sound Medicine. The Prime

John Mills

APPENDIX C

My Communication to Kaua`i HealthCare Providers
and
For all Patients scheduling a Consultation with me

A model for reinventing yourself and designing your role in the
communities you serve— expressing yourself exactly how you wish
to show up

John C Mills MD
Blending the Best of East & West

Aloha to all HealthCare Providers and Practitioners on Kaua'i

This letter serves as an introduction to my practice for those of you who don't know me, and to familiarize you with my professional background and my long history in HealthCare, wellness work and wellness education.

Briefly, I am a fully trained Orthopaedic surgeon who then shifted into a long career in Emergency Medicine, for the purpose of owning a schedule I could work with as I raised my family of five children, be available to them as they grew up, always a part of their lives, and manage work hours more on my calling than is afforded in a private practice—this worked very well and taught me the extraordinary value of family closeness and family love.

Simultaneous with this I spent a career in the military on both Active Duty and Active Reserve Duty, retiring from the military after 30 years. This combined military service, and a civilian medical practice taught me much, and both were great experiences.

Always, I maintained a Holistic perspective and an interest in examining what creates a state of superb wellbeing, vitality, and contentment. This led me down a path combining East and West philosophies of health and healing, as well as an energetic approach to healing pathways.

It is no longer my calling to see patients only in a traditional medical clinical setting, care dictated in my experience by a system which falls short of the optimal expectations of many patients and healthcare providers alike.

So, what is next for me is an expanding interest in the field of wellness, looking together at what it takes to create a mental, emotional, physical condition way beyond merely the absence of disease. On the following pages is a glimpse of my background.

This communication is simply to say aloha, to make you aware of what I offer, to learn more about your practices as you wish to share, and to be available to you and your patients or clients in any way I may be of service to you.

You may ask what exactly am I offering to you by way of any referral you may be considering?

Throughout all my years of practice in a variety of clinical settings, one of the things I valued most was my relationship with other practitioners I could trust and always rely on for sound advice when I needed it—a colleague who would join me in providing optimal comprehensive care of my patients when I wanted another experienced source to consult, to communicate knowledge and ideas that would further my patient's recovery or desired health goals.

In short, I am available to assist with any patient, perhaps in particular, your difficult ones in which you'd like an interested colleague to render some thoughts, given my background in western medicine (Orthopaedic Surgery, Emergency Medicine, and Holistic Wellness), and my experience in eastern and energetic principles of health and healing as well.

I will be seeing patients in an office setting in Kapaa owned by Dr Carrie 'Karu' Hodder LAc MAcOM, Chinese Medicine & Acupuncture, at Feel Better Kauai, 4569 Kukui Street, Suite 201, Kapaa, HI 96746. For those whom it is more convenient, I will offer appointments out of my home office on the South Shore in Koloa.

Please see my attached professional background and list of services, an About Me page, and some additional information—a website is currently in the design stage. I am more than happy to answer any questions you may have and work with you in any capacity that we design together in the care of your patients or clients, or anyone else you may wish to refer.

Looking forward to working with you.

In Health, John Mills

PROFESSIONAL BACKGROUND

JOHN C MILLS MD

YALE UNIVERSITY SCHOOL OF MEDICINE

SURGICAL RESIDENCIES AT YALE AND TUFTS

ORTHOPAEDIC SURGEON

EMERGENCY MEDICINE PHYSICIAN

HOLISTIC PRACTITIONER

HEALTH & WELLNESS

ENERGY MEDICINE

SHAMAN

AYURVEDIC PRACTITIONER

YOGA INSTRUCTOR RYT-500

WILDERNESS MEDICINE

RETIRED COLONEL US ARMY SPECIAL FORCES

VETERANS HEALTH

BLENDING THE BEST OF EAST AND WEST

TOPICS FOR DISCUSSION OR WORKSHOPS

All Currently Offered and Designed to Meet your Needs

FOCUS ON WELLNESS Discussion Series: A series of discussions designed to enrich our experience of Life:

1) Getting Well, Staying Well, Feeling Great;
2) Living Wellness;
3) The Natural Nutritional Mind, Body, Spirit Path to Health, Happiness, Enlightenment, and Weight Loss;
4) Health, Wealth and Love

NATURE AND YOU Program: A discussion and workshop designed to increase our awareness of, and our relationship with, Nature

LET'S TALK ABOUT HEALTH, FOR OURSELVES, FOR OUR PLANET: A blending of Eastern and Western teachings and philosophy, Energetic Principles, and a Mind-Body-Spirit approach to Health and Well-Being

THE PATH OF YOGA

MINDFUL STRETCHING FOR INJURY PREVENTION

THE AYURVEDIC DISCUSSION SERIES:

1) Introduction to Ayurveda;
2) The Ayurvedic Approach to Diet and Lifestyle;

3) Yoga and Ayurveda, an Integrative Approach

YOGA, AYURVEDA AND SPIRIT

ENERGY MEDICINE AND QUANTUM THEORY (Made Simple)

TO YOUR HEALTH . . . A WORK OF ART, A WORK OF FICTION

THE VALUE OF MOVEMENT, PLAY AND SPIRIT

VIBRANT HEALTH FOR HEALTH CARE PROFESSIONALS

ASK THE DOCTOR

BUSINESS/CORPORATE/SCHOOL/HOSPITAL WELLNESS PROGRAM

DEEPENING INTUITION

CREATING A LIFE OF PURPOSE—AND LOVING IT!!!

REDESIGNING YOURSELF

PLANETARY STEWARDSHIP and THE FLYING WARRIOR TRAINING PROGRAM

THE PATH OF THE SHAMAN

www.ingramcontent.com/pod-product-compliance
Lightning Source LLC
Chambersburg PA
CBHW050239270326
41914CB00041BA/2040/J